T0327737

INTERNET CURES

The Social Lives of Digital Miracles

Dang Nguyen

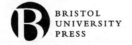
BRISTOL
UNIVERSITY
PRESS

First published in Great Britain in 2025 by

Bristol University Press
University of Bristol
1–9 Old Park Hill
Bristol
BS2 8BB
UK
t: +44 (0)117 374 6645
e: bup-info@bristol.ac.uk

Details of international sales and distribution partners are available at bristoluniversitypress.co.uk

© Bristol University Press 2025

British Library Cataloguing in Publication Data
A catalogue record for this book is available from the British Library

ISBN 978-1-5292-3516-6 hardcover
ISBN 978-1-5292-3517-3 ePub
ISBN 978-1-5292-3518-0 ePdf

The right of Dang Nguyen to be identified as author of this work has been asserted by her in accordance with the Copyright, Designs and Patents Act 1988.

Cover design: Nicky Borowiec
Front cover image: Getty Images/Luis Diaz Devesa
Bristol University Press uses environmentally responsible print partners.
Printed and bound in Great Britain by CPI Group (UK) Ltd, Croydon, CR0 4YY

FSC
www.fsc.org
MIX
Paper | Supporting
responsible forestry
FSC® C013604

For Tammie

Contents

List of Figures and Tables

Figures

Tables

About the Author

Dang Nguyen is Research Fellow in the ARC Centre of Excellence for Automated Decision-Making and Society at RMIT University, Australia. She researches the social implications of digital technologies by bringing together methods of different disciplines and traditions – and by looking beyond Western contexts. Dang is the author of *Digital Research Methods and the Diaspora: Assembling Transnational Networks with and beyond Digital Data* (Routledge, 2023). Currently based in Australia, Dang was born and raised in Vietnam and continues to conduct research into Vietnam and the South East Asian region more generally.

Acknowledgements

I wish to thank Michael Arnold for allowing me to plant the first seeds of what would eventually become this book, all the way back in 2018 in Melbourne. I owe a debt of gratitude to my mentors at Yale, Erik Harms and Emily Erikson, for their intellectual generosity and collegiality during my time there, which was formative for the writing of much of this project. Julian Thomas and the TCP Lab team convinced me that I can, and should, write this book; I thank them for being the intellectual support network I didn't know I deserve.

Finally, I wish to thank Paul Stevens for the care and trust he places in this project; without his vision for what a book could be, this book would simply not be possible.

1

Introduction: Of Internet Cures and Digital Miracles

Among the many plotlines that made up the story of the COVID-19 pandemic, that of miracle cures dominated early on. While Australians were panic buying toilet rolls and Americans hand sanitizers and face masks (Meyersohn, 2020; Stratton, 2021), across South East Asia people were nervously looking for ways to protect themselves by turning to familiar wisdom. Cure-alls and self-concocted remedies for COVID-19 soon circulated on the Vietnamese internet; they included practices such as consuming boiled lemongrass and orange zest before entering or leaving the house, massaging medicated oil onto the feet before bedtime, incorporating spices like chilli, ginger, and garlic into daily meals, or using a hairdryer to blow hot air along the spine and toes (Nguyen, 2020). Similarly, Cambodian YouTube recommended drinking boiled garlic juice, sunbathing in intense heat, or applying garlic juice to the nose to boost one's immune system, thus warding off the virus (Nguyen, 2020). In Indonesia, the demand for turmeric and ginger skyrocketed as they are essential ingredients in the traditional *jamu* herbal drink (which the Indonesian president endorsed for boosting the immune system and protecting against COVID-19) – leading to soaring prices for these plants (The Straits Times, 2020).

In Malaysia, dried ginseng, scallops, and sea cucumber were in demand as ingredients for *tong sui*, a traditional Chinese sweet warm soup believed to boost immunity (Chandran, 2020). In Thailand, bitter-tasting *kariyat* was promoted as an effective treatment of coronavirus symptoms, while the Department of Thai Traditional Medicine and Government Pharmaceutical Organization were working on the development of COVID-19 cures using the medicinal herb *Andrographis paniculate*, with inconclusive results (The Nation Thailand, 2020). In a similar vein, the Philippine Council on Health Research and Development of the Department of Science and Technology was reported to research coconut oil as a potential agent against the virus (Lim, 2020). South East Asian states were not alone in aspiring to develop treatments for COVID-19 by drawing on knowledge paradigms closely bound in nationalistic sentiments about culture and tradition. To the north, China advocated for 'Chinese solutions' to the pandemic and sharing 'Chinese experience' in the form of a 'lung-cleansing and detoxifying soup' distributed in Wuhan hospitals (Gan and Xiong, 2020). China's National Health Commission also endorsed injections that contain bear bile powder as treatment, to the dismay of critics (Fobar, 2020).

The resurgence of indigenous non-biomedical practices fuelled by peer-to-peer information circulating on social media platforms, however, long preceded the pandemic. To be sure, non-biomedical practices – therapeutic modalities that exist alongside but never in isolation from scientific biomedicine – never ceased to exist across the South East Asian region and its neighbour in the north. Although colonial powers invariably marginalized and stigmatized indigenous forms of therapy throughout the region during the 20th century, these treatments remain widely practised – a result of insufficient reach and investment of resources from colonial governments as much as the allure of traditional cures. Post-colonial governments across South East Asia also variously co-opt, scientize, and revitalize medical traditions as part of their nation-building projects (Wahlberg, 2006; Monnais et al, 2011; Monnais, 2019). In mid-1950s China, Mao Tse-Tung went back on his revolutionary position against traditional medical practitioners after comparing them to 'circus entertainers, snake oil salesmen, and street hawkers' and declared traditional Chinese medicine to be cultivated and celebrated as a 'national treasure' (Harrington, 2008, p 225). That non-biomedical recipes proliferate on social media and that emergent non-biomedical practices evolve alongside new mediated modes of communication is but the latest episode of this long, tumultuous medical history.

A theoretical interlude

I became interested in studying internet cures in 2017, when the research agenda around misinformation was taking shape after the election of Donald Trump in the US. There was a marked uptick in research interests around the role of misinformation in political campaigns and its potential impact on electoral outcomes; scholars, journalists, and researchers from various disciplines became very invested in understanding the spread of misinformation, its sources, and its effects on public opinion. The idea that our information environment was being flooded with rubbish information – which adversely impacted our information diet – turned out to be a very potent idea. Soon enough, media organizations, technology companies, and policy makers also engaged in efforts to understand and address the challenges posed by misinformation, resulting in collaborations between researchers and various stakeholders. Tools and techniques were being developed to detect and counteract misinformation; fact-checking initiatives started to gain prominence as news organizations, universities, and social media platforms worked together to debunk false claims and verify the accuracy of political statements (Cerone et al, 2020; Juneja and Mitra, 2022). A strong research agenda around assessing the effectiveness of interventions, such as providing corrective information or making tweaks to platform design to mitigate the impact of misinformation, was also taking shape. Research into parsing the motivations and strategies of those creating and disseminating misinformation, including political actors, foreign entities, and individual users, also quickly became cemented as a staple in the agenda, drawing on well-established programmes in political science research (Swire et al, 2017; Li, 2020; Nunziato, 2020).

Amid this burgeoning landscape of research, health misinformation research was also taking shape. If we were really living in an era of 'fake news' (Wang et al, 2019b), it seemed reasonable to assume that political misinformation was not the only form of misinformation that we got exposed to. If anything, the consequences of health misinformation could be so much more dire: health is a matter of literal life and death. In a systematic literature review on health misinformation on social media, Wang et al (2019b, p 1) remarked: 'In democracies where ideas compete in the marketplace for attention, accurate scientific information, which may be difficult to comprehend and even dull, is easily crowded out by sensationalized news.' The stakes could not be higher: not only was democracy at risk, but science was also under attack. The social media genie was out of the bottle, and we are now left to navigate the treacherous landscape of misinformation and restore trust in our institutions.

This book is an attempt at complicating these narratives, which have rapidly become crystallized around the notion of 'misinformation warfare', where researchers become ordained as critical agents in untangling the intricate web of deceptive tactics, uncovering the truth, and shedding light on the complexities of information manipulation. To be clear, the research programme that came out of these dominant narratives is crucial to bringing the social sciences and humanities into the project of defining and addressing the most important issues of our time; that misinformation has become a common object with which different academic disciplines could engage and collaborate is a remarkable achievement. The goal of this book is neither to reinvent nor debunk misinformation research. Its goal, rather, is to enrich the misinformation research agenda by infusing the notion of misinformation with history and culture – while taking the technologies that co-constitute this phenomenon seriously. This task requires the development of new language, as well as the eclectic use of methods that might not otherwise usually accompany one another.

To this end, a few terminology clarifications are in order. 'Internet cures' as used in this book refers to both the proliferation of cure-alls and folk remedies that animated the previous pages and the empirical reality that the internet and digital technologies are where many people turn to for solutions to various problems, challenges, or ailments. More than just a technical system that transmits data around the world, the internet has a distinct palliative function in our society. 'Digital miracles' refers to the ways in which people assign unprecedented and almost miraculous qualities to digital technologies and their transformative potential. It captures the perception that these technologies possess extraordinary powers to revolutionize and solve a multitude of complex issues across different domains – including health and illness. Non-biomedical knowledge – or non-biomedical modalities – has its own dedicated chapter (Chapter 3). As a concept, non-biomedical knowledge is better equipped to capture the diversity as well as the historical continuities and discontinuities of therapeutic traditions and practices at the margin of mainstream scientific medicine – compared to a range of existing, often conflated terms such as traditional medicine, alternative medicine, unorthodox medicine, and so on.

Let's contextualize this with a story from the field. When Quang, a Vietnamese American living in Orange County, California (Chapters 6 and 7), learned that he was diagnosed with advanced prostate cancer, he decided that it was time for him and his family to return to Vietnam for the first time in 46 years. Like many Vietnamese refugees who successfully built a new life in the US at the end of the Vietnam War, Quang's voluntary exile from mainland Vietnam was motivated in large part by the political conviction that to return to mainland Vietnam is to concede to the legitimacy of the current government. Having made the decision to forego chemotherapy in the US, Quang had been relying on *diện chẩn* – an emerging non-biomedical method that involves the use of spiky tools to massage various points on the face to cure ailments – to manage his condition. Quang was introduced to *diện chẩn* (transliterally 'face diagnosis') by a family member, who had learned about this method from a friend practising it on clients at a Vietnamese spa. Having located a Facebook group led by followers of the method in Vietnam, Quang would tune into the group's livestreaming sessions daily to watch the method being practised on people who sought treatment for various diseases and conditions, as well as practising along to the group's livestreamed tutorials. Because of his prostate cancer, Quang practised along to tutorials that focused on six particular zones on the face that supposedly correspond to the lymphoid system in the body, according to the *diện chẩn* method. Starting with rubbing and pressing on various mapped out points on the face, Quang slowly transitioned to using specialized spiky tools – acquired by his wife via her contact in Vietnam – to roll across these points for better accuracy and pressure. He regularly shared with the online group how *diện chẩn* supported him during both good and bad days, occasionally engaging in video calls with group leaders to personalize treatment plans. At first, the rubs and rolls caused discomfort, especially when he encountered specific acupressure points. Over time, as Quang's techniques improved, he noticed that practising the method alleviated his urination and back pain – something he had not expected to happen. Convinced that *diện chẩn* held the key to his cancer cure, Quang took a leap of faith and flew his family back to Ho Chi Minh City to meet Bùi Quốc Châu, the progenitor of the method. Digital miracles akin to Quang's remarkable journey happen every day; this book is an attempt at understanding them.

The book takes a mixed methods approach to assembling networks of digital miracles. It draws extensively on the vocabulary of Actor-Network Theory (ANT), a sociological framework that emphasizes the interconnectedness of human and non-human actors in shaping social phenomena (Latour, 2005). Central to ANT is the insight that actor-networks are accomplishments that must be explained rather than assumed; actions are therefore always *overtaken* by actors – the idea that actions or intentions attributed to human actors are not solely determined by their individual agency, but are shaped and influenced by the network of relationships in which they are embedded. A network mediates and influences the actions and intentions of individual actors, often in ways that may go beyond their initial intentions or expectations; human and non-human agency is therefore relational and distributed. To assemble a network of digital miracles is to recognize and enlist the different entities that contribute to not only the enactment of digital miracles, but also the *situations* of this enactment. A task of this nature requires both the interpretive-theoretical and ethical perspectives from the social sciences and the analytical capabilities of computational methods. To this end, the book combines computational mapping (drawing from social media data collected from 2014 to 2018) and ethnographic accounts (collected from 2018 to 2020 across Vietnam and the US). By adopting this hybrid approach, the book assembles how the social lives of non-biomedical knowledge are enacted as sympoietic systems. Sympoietic systems circulate without a central authority or underlying coherence; they assume autonomous and divergent paths, existing with multiple temporalities that contribute to their continuous yet episodic evolution.

To the extent that non-biomedical knowledge is *not* misinformation, it has a much longer *durée*, persisting beyond the rise and fall of scientific paradigms. A well-studied example of this is American mind-body medicine, whose narratives are rooted in the Bible and other religious writings that describe the struggle against 'possession' by demonic forces (Harrington, 2008). Belief in demonic possession and its exorcism by priests was widely held in various cultures worldwide and remained an integral aspect of Catholic theology – largely unchanged – until the beginning of the 21st century. Harrington

(2008) identified six narratives of mind–body medicine that traces the historical evolution of more or less the same idea: that the body is a mindful entity. These narratives are the power of suggestion (a narrative that science developed to explain cases in which an authority figure, whether a priest uttering incantations or a doctor administering a placebo, cures afflictions that may have no organic cause), the body that speaks (the scientific quest for nonphysical causes of patients' symptoms and cures outside of chemical pills and surgical procedures), the power of positive thinking (Christian Science and its modern frequent dialogue with the biomedical profession), broken by modern life (Cold War era narrative on stress and trauma, and experiences of malaise), healing ties (social cohesion as prophylactic, if not the cure, for cancer), and Eastward journeys (orientalist conceptions of the wise 'Other', whose therapeutic treasures are beyond those imaginable to the West). The non-biomedical modalities discussed in this book are similarly practices that have carved out their own space, coexisting alongside and co-opting scientific biomedical advancements.

This book investigates how the practice and reception of non-biomedical modalities have evolved in response to digital technologies by examining the emergence of new hybrid analogue–digital forms of these cures. These hybrids encompass a wide range of format: from photographs of hand-written miracle recipes to machine-readable transcriptions shared as Facebook posts, from video tutorials demonstrating miracle cures to one-on-one healing sessions conducted over livestreaming platforms. At the surface level, technology is enabling the digital codification of existing bodies of miraculous folk medicine by migrating our dominant written culture to social media. On a deeper level, technology also enables emergent non-biomedical practices with and through rich media such as video streaming and livestreaming. The digital miracles that unfold on these dynamic and interactive media, where healers claim to cure their patients from a distance in real time, follow a distinct logic of digital play – as the book will show. By contextualizing non-biomedical cures within their lived realities, we can understand the enduring and ongoing nature of these practices. Their intersection with digital technologies is the latest instalment in a long-standing history of continual but episodic evolution.

Among the first of its kind to combine computational mapping and ethnographic research to study internet cures, the book takes an analytical approach to explore the worlds that miracle cures as living practices facilitate through their interaction with new technologies. It aims to fill the gap between two main currents of social research on folk medicine and non-biomedical practices: epistemological approaches (emphasizing these modalities' relationship to Science Proper) and health communication approaches (emphasizing their persuasion as worldviews and cultural expressions in online and offline contexts). It also aims to recast internet cures as diasporic practices that are entangled in existing and emerging networks of materiality and ideas. As such, the core contribution of the book is in proposing new ways of thinking about internet cures through dissemination of original empirical research.

The kind of study done in this book is not without history, however. This book is the latest addition to a broader movement in research that commits to a new and progressive form of quali-quantitative methods, which Blok and Pedersen (2014) call 'complementary social science'. Complementary social science stitches together data worlds produced through computational and ethnographic methods, so that researchers can look at established concepts such as 'personhood', 'politics', or 'the social' in ways that are more responsive to the mutual shaping of humans and non-humans. Antecedents to complementary social science include long-standing movements within Science and Technology Studies and related disciplines in which largely qualitative researchers have been adopting and adapting quantitative tools to their own ends (Callon et al, 1986; Latour et al, 1992; Rogers and Marres, 2000). Latour et al (2012) revisited Gabriel Tardes' monads by working quantitatively and qualitatively with digital datasets, arguing for a navigational research practice that modifies social theory in radical ways. Many recent studies employed approaches similar to the one employed in this book: Laaksonen et al (2017), for example, employed what they called 'big-data-augmented online ethnography' to study candidate–candidate interaction during elections in Finland. Ruckenstein (2019) explored human–drug associations using Medicine Radar, a computational tool that allows her to raise questions about the ways a digital device pushes us to rethink how drugs are known in the everyday. Munk (2019) assembled the new Nordic food movement on the web using a range of quali-quantitative methods, while Moats (2021) argued that researchers stand to benefit from seeing knowledge production as a shared and ongoing problem across disciplines through reflections across Science and Technology Studies (STS), medical sociology, medicine, media studies, and anthropology.

This book is one of the first few book-length responses to a larger movement in research which assembles its research phenomenon by means of both computational and qualitative methods. However, insofar as there is an explicit concern with theorizing, this book is also a philosophical book. The kind of philosophy that this book commits to follows a long-standing tradition in STS to move philosophy away from formats that carry universalistic pretentions, but that in fact hide the locality to which they pertain. The book is explicit about its local, albeit dispersed, origins: throughout the book, there are snapshot stories about Vietnamese miracle cures assembled through computational and ethnographic analyses. The book takes its cue from STS classics, such as Annemarie Mol's theorization of the body through fieldwork conducted in a large university hospital in a medium-sized Dutch town about the atherosclerosis disease of the leg arteries (Mol, 2002), or Bruno Latour and Steve Woolgar's theorization of the construction of scientific fact by following and talking to scientists and engineers at The Salk Institute for Biological Studies (Latour and Woolgar, 1986). The idea here, however, is not to celebrate localism instead of universalism. Instead, the aim is to keep track as persistently as possible of what it is that alters when digital miracles travel from one place to another.

Previews

The book is organized in three parts. Part I contextualizes the various terminologies introduced here – internet cures, digital miracles, and non-biomedical knowledge – both as *in vivo* concepts in Vietnamese vernacular and as theoretical concepts that travel beyond their situated meanings. Chapter 2 presents Vietnam as a site of empirical work; this empirical site is understood not as a unitary nation-state, but as ongoing enactments of shared identity, common meaning, and bounded sovereignty that can be traced and assembled. In Vietnam, the notion of the miracle cure is historically tied not to a Christian divine intervention tradition, but rather to the miraculous healing effects of the everyday garden and jungle herbs and plants. Miraculous family recipes of Southern medicine were systematically documented and codified firstly by *Tuệ Tĩnh*, a 14th-century physician known as *Thánh thuốc Nam* (Saint of Southern medicine), and later on by *Hải Thượng Lãn Ông*, who was honoured as the Great Herb Doctor (*Đại Y Tông*), in the 18th century. The authority of the traditional healer – sometimes touted under the titles of 'miraculous doctors' (*thần y*) or 'doctors of good conscience' (*lương y*) – persists well into the digital age, with social media groups being formed around these figures. Southern medicine (*thuốc Nam*) is usually associated with empirical domestic medicine, where secret family recipes are usually shared for a fee or passed along as gifts among friends. Northern medicine (*thuốc Bắc*) is usually associated with a more learned and advanced tradition of the 'North' – in this case, referring to an ancient Sino-Vietnamese civilization that existed prior to Southern colonization of the Cham and the Khmer (modern central and Southern Vietnam). As the West conceived the East as a foil to its own Western values and lifestyles in an inversion where the East had to become the spiritual, moral, and medical exemplar from which the West has much to learn, the East never quite existed as a coherent monolith. There is often cross-pollination, exchange of ideas, and incorporation of practices from different branches and traditions; where synergies exist, integrative approaches that draw from multiple knowledge systems tend to emerge.

Chapter 3 presents an empirically grounded argument for the term non-biomedical modalities through a large-scale co-word analysis of the disparate literatures on traditional medicine, herbal medicine, alternative and complementary medicine, unorthodox cures, and unconventional medicine. As a theoretical gesture, this exercise uses formal analysis to capture the historical disruption that biomedicine both as a scientific discipline and as a mechanism of body surveillance came to solidify modernity around the world. The analysis also highlights the continuity of medical practices that persist at the margin of the scientific enterprise as they continue to evolve and transform themselves through their interaction with biomedicine. True to the ANT approach, this analysis sees knowledge production as problematic socio-cognitive networks of hybrid communities, whose interests are aggregated and funnelled through translations of scientific publications as literary inscriptions (Callon et al, 1983). Translation as well as counter-translation of and by relevant actors make network associations possible; within this framework, words as they are positioned and stabilized within literary inscriptions act as translation operators that allow actors to navigate and consolidate webs of interests. Keywords and terminologies as translation operators can reveal poles of interest, their convergence or intersection, relationships that are developed around them, and the general configuration of the knowledge network.

Part II explores the migration of our dominant written culture to social media, and how this migration has enabled the codification and digitization of traditional healing recipes from different Vietnamese medical traditions. Once kept within families of traditional medical doctors through oral traditions or written up on paper and sold for a fee, these recipes are now shared, discussed, and debated across social media networks on a much larger scale. The ready computability of the written text is a symptom of our writing society, one that is saturated with traces of written objects. Chapter 4 explores the crowd digitization of healing recipes and the digitality of writing by presenting an anatomy of these recipes on social media, whose form and format are contingent on platform affordances. The chapter also reflects on the automated process of collecting the computed texts in these recipes, their executable nature which renders them amenable to a plethora of automated data manipulation, measuring, and analysis techniques, and what these analyses can and cannot say about these texts. That the task of meaning-making from letters and numbers is so readily computable – compared to the still and moving images, for example – says something about the relationship between the written text and computability. Computational analyses can be mobilized to say something new about texts and networks of texts, to make formal observations about not only what these texts mean, but also the relationships between them.

Chapter 5 presents a computational analysis of the network characteristics of, and discourses present within, three popular Vietnamese non-biomedical knowledge Facebook sites over a period of five years. These large-scale datasets are studied using social network analysis and generative statistical models for topic analysis (Latent Dirichlet allocation). Forty-nine unique topics were quantitatively identified and qualitatively interpreted. Although non-biomedical networks on Facebook are growing both in terms of scale and popularity, sub-network comment activities within these networks exhibit 'small world' characteristics. When a network exhibits 'small world' characteristics, there is efficient information dissemination within these networks; they are also robust to node failures. The analysis presented in this chapter suggests that social media seem to be replicating existing social dynamics that historically enable the maintenance of traditional forms of medical knowledge, rather than transforming them.

Part III turns to emergent dynamic technologies, such as livestreaming, and explores how these technologies bring with them new temporal and spatial sensibilities of therapy. Insofar as Part III is in conversation with Part II, it interrogates the conditions of possibility for digital miracles, while Part II takes for granted that digitality is a vehicle for miracle cures. Chapter 6 explores the practice of livestreaming miracle healing on social media by examining what this practice is doing to experiences of downtime during episodes of illness and personal crises. It draws on fieldwork conducted in Vietnam and the US on the transnational practices of *diện chẩn* (literally 'face diagnosis'), an emergent Vietnamese non-biomedical practice that claims to diagnose and treat most diseases through particular ways to massage the face. Particularly, different constellations of points on a human face, according to *diện chẩn*, are said to correspond to different organs in the human body. If these points are massaged correctly, the claim is that any and all diseases within the corresponding organs can be cured. This chapter interrogates enactments of liveness through social media livestreaming as oscillating between simultaneity and instantaneity; it argues that this oscillation allows for downtime to be recuperated, and for tactile explorations of technology and the body not only to overcome boredom, but also to facilitate self-maintenance of the body.

Chapter 7 explores practices of digital miracles as digital play, with a particular focus on the construction of imaginary digital situations with and through technology. Drawing from the same fieldwork presented in Chapter 6, this chapter explores the ways in which technology is understood as interface and inscrutable systems that enters the everyday world of human actors to perform in magical ways. Particularly, this chapter explores magical claims made by Bùi Quốc Châu, the inventor of the *diện chẩn* method, of curing patients via digital technology. Châu, through very elaborate (though misguided) articulations of digital technologies, sees the internet as a medium that allows him to employ quasi-physical magical powers to intervene on the conditions of his patients who live overseas. This chapter connects this domain of magic-making with play: magic, which sets an ideal standard, is not to be approached in reality, yet practical technical action can be oriented towards it. Following anthropologist Alfred Gell, this chapter explores how when Châu claims to force 'internal energy' out through his palms over his phone screen while narrating the impact of his actions on the patients he is curing, he is doing the same thing as a child transforming themselves into an airplane (with arms extended, and the appropriate sound effects and swooping movements) while providing a continuous stream of commentary on their own behaviour (for example, now I am doing this, now I am doing that, and now this will happen …).

Together, the chapters in this book put forward a theoretically imaginative, historically considered, and methodologically pragmatic account of internet cures as world-making and world-affirming. The book seeks not to have 'the last word' on the subject matter; rather, it wishes to open up new avenues of research, new conversations, and new ways of looking at therapeutic practices that continue to persist alongside scientific practices. Any social research purporting to shine light on how the internet is shaping our individual and collective well-being cannot afford to dismissively ignore non-biomedical practices both in their *longue durée* and emergent enactments.

PART I

Contextualizing Internet Cures and Digital Miracles

Prologue: Miracles before the digital

Miracle cures differ greatly across time and context. What all miracle cures share, however, is their being unusual and unexpected from the perspective of empirical scientific knowledge – where an effect is said to have happened despite the absence of an acceptable cause. The miracle cure is both an *in vivo* concept in vernacular language and a theoretical category that travels far beyond their situated meanings. In Vietnam, the notion of the miracle cure (*thần dược*) is historically tied not to a Christian divine intervention tradition, but rather to the miraculous healing effects of much of the everyday garden and jungle herbs and plants. By recasting miracle cures as non-biomedical modalities, whose processes of producing, propagating, and living are historical and ongoing, we can begin to discern the limits of the misinformation paradigm and interrogate these modalities as both mediated and material.

Miracle Cures in Context: Vietnam as Research Site

What constitutes an appropriate site for empirical research? A research site limits what can be feasibly studied, especially given constraints on time and resources, and shapes the usefulness of the empirical work in relation to other past and future research. Yet research sites are not naturally occurring, ready-made fields of events that are easily accessible to researchers. Morita (2020) remarks that growing interest in the multiplicity of knowledge practices in the non-West has illuminated complex arrangements of difference that require new vocabulary beyond that of 'culture' and 'society' as autonomous entities. In imagining multiplicity, researchers make the movements and connections that explain not a world that exists 'out there', but rather problematize problem spaces in which a situation becomes a problem as it recursively refers to descriptions of itself.

As such, Vietnam as a country, a culture, a society is not a self-evident social context in which researchers can readily 'immerse' or unproblematically interrogate. What makes Vietnam appropriate as a research site is through the ongoing enactments of shared identity, common meaning, and bounded sovereignty that can be traced and assembled. Vietnam is both a site and a case insofar as it is well-circumscribed enough to not hide its locality while offering itself as points of contrast, reference, or comparison for other sites and situations. The locale of this book is local, albeit dispersed; while it seeks to do away with scholarly formats that carry universalistic pretentions, it is worth reiterating that the point is not to favour localism over universalism. A carefully studied case allows us to unravel what remains the same and what changes from one situation to the next, and thus informs findings that are particular to situations and findings that are not.

In circumscribing a case study as an ongoing enactment of sociality, we are preparing ourselves to attend to events that may disrupt and unfasten any preconceived notion about social relations. In doing this, we should also be open to the possibility of being taken by the actors involved to unfamiliar territories. What is at stake here is not only the changed 'cosmos' of social realities before and after experiences of illness as disruptive bodily events, but also the transnational social relations being mediatized by technologies – that which renders Vietnam as multiple, beyond its geographic sovereignty.

Much like social normalcy, once unbuttoned, contexts and locations are vulnerable to uncertainty, contingency, and change (Schillmeier, 2014). In committing to unsettling any static notion about what Vietnam is and could become, I have made the analytical decision to render Vietnam as unfinished, open, and plural – in keeping with a processual and dynamic outlook to the history of places. This will prove to be particularly fruitful in Part III, as we explore the distributed nature of mediatized spatiality and temporality in livestreaming digital miracles across the Vietnamese diaspora. For now, let us turn our attention to the context of digital Vietnam and how this context colours our understanding of miracle cures.

The emergence of digital Vietnam

In 2023, 79.1 per cent of the population in Vietnam (around 77.93 million people) were using the internet – higher than the Asia-Pacific average at 53.6 per cent (Internet World Stats, 2023; Kemp, 2023). The majority of internet users in Vietnam access the internet via mobile broadband, with 82.7 million mobile broadband subscriptions recorded in 2022 (MIC, 2023). Vietnamese are increasingly performing significant parts of their everyday lives online; the average daily time spent on the internet is 6.23 hours, 2.32 of which are spent on social media (Kemp, 2023). Facebook is the third most popular website in Vietnam after Google and YouTube and is the most popular social media platform in the country (Kemp, 2023). There are around 66.2 million Facebook users in Vietnam in 2023, making Vietnam the seventh-largest market for Facebook worldwide (Kemp, 2023; We Are Social, 2023). This intense participation in digital modes of sociality is having significant impacts on the way in which Vietnamese seek, construct, produce, and consume information about their social world.

Emerging modes of digital sociality are crucial to the formation of the Vietnamese digital diaspora. The availability of digital technologies at low cost, together with increasingly widespread internet adoption, has allowed diasporic groups to deepen the quality of ties being forged and maintained with their country of origin. This deepening of quality is thanks to increases in frequency and intensity of diasporic communication, made possible as a result of both fundamental changes in the structure of mediated communication and thus the communication environment at large, as well as the emergence of new possibilities of diaspora enactment thanks to the media-rich characteristics of the internet. A Vietnamese American struggling with a terminal medical condition in California might not only find community, but also tangible support, on Facebook groups based in Vietnam. Increasingly, due to the dynamic intensification of these digital connections, the functioning of digital diasporas also transforms beyond merely maintaining ethnic identities and cultural bonds.

Nedelcu (2019) argued that transformations of diasporic functioning can be mapped against three main aspects: the actualization of the homeland as memory on a day-to-day basis, the replacement of diaspora as 'non-lieu' by a sense of shared virtual place, and the agency capability of acting transnationally in real-time. In this light, digital diaspora is not only a new enactment of diaspora, but also becomes an expression of the cosmopolitan condition. Digital formations facilitate and transform the very possibilities for diasporic affiliation; digital diaspora as space is therefore dynamic, processual, relational, and contingent. Digital diaspora is articulated as fluid and relational because what it means to enact diasporas has changed by means of engagement with technology: processes of becoming diasporan are increasingly subject to ever-more complex articulations and negotiations, and with them come new configurations of participation and identification. While maintaining a well-established orientation towards notions of homeland, origin culture, and senses of belonging, these new configurations are enmeshed in other networks of practice that make the diasporic experience increasingly elastic. It might not occur to a traditional healer who has spent all his life in Vietnam to take on clients overseas until various livestreaming and videocall technologies become readily available in the palm of his hand, making it possible – and sometimes necessary – to enroll in a digital diasporic network that transforms the very nature of his practice.

These emerging configurations are also historically contingent. The emergence of digital Vietnam can hardly be understood in separation from the more foundational developments in digital infrastructure and its associated geopolitics. In the case of Vietnam, its historical entanglements with China tend to translate to a convergence of digital governance strategies, where Vietnamese policies and practices often draw inspiration from Chinese models while concurrently asserting its own cultural and political autonomy. Commentators have long remarked on the similarities between the way in which Vietnam and China approach internet regulation (OpenNet Initiative, 2012; AFP, 2019; Sherman, 2019); most recently, Vietnam has been a notable recipient of Chinese government funding through the 'Two Corridors, One Belt' initiative and the Belt and Road Initiative (BRI). There are distinct parallels between the way in which issues such as internet censorship, data governance, and internet surveillance play out across these contexts, such that the cultural and political entanglements between the two countries continue well into the digital age. Patterns of resistance, cooperation, co-option, and compromise between the two countries can be found over and over again across different domains of life; a prime example of this is in the history of indigenous Vietnamese medicine.

Material entanglements: a short history of medical traditions in Vietnam

Entanglements between Vietnam and China also manifest themselves materially. The first imperial power to carry out a 'civilizing mission' in Vietnam, China claimed to have endowed the 'unenlightened' people of Vietnam with agriculture, writing, and medicine – a trio of gifts that French colonists later took credit for modernizing (Thompson, 2015). Han census of AD 2 and manuscripts unearthed in southern China, however, show that early Vietnamese appear to have been well acquainted with all three. Agriculture was well developed in Vietnam before the arrival of the Chinese; the Viet had medical lore well suited to their local conditions, and although Vietnamese wrote many of their texts in Classical Chinese before the adoption of the modern Vietnamese alphabetic script *quốc ngữ*, a fully functional Vietnamese writing system was developed around the time the Vietnamese regained independence from China in 939 CE – a language called *Nôm*, meaning 'Southern characters' (Thompson, 2015). The majority of surviving Vietnamese medical texts are written in either *Nôm* or *Hán-Nôm* (a mixture of both Classical Chinese and *Nôm* scripts). This refutes the common misperception that Vietnamese used *Nôm* only to write literature, while using Chinese to write everything else (Thompson, 2015).

These finer historical points matter because the relationship between medicine and writing/language in Vietnam is that of a complex nature: in Vietnamese vernacular, Vietnamese medicine has always been understood in relation to what it is not (Monnais et al, 2011). Traditional medicine in Vietnam is divided into two main branches: Northern medicine (*thuốc Bắc*), referring to Chinese-inspired medicine, and Southern medicine (*thuốc Nam*), referring to indigenous Vietnamese medicine. The word *Bắc* (which literally means North) also refers to China and all things Chinese, in the same way that *Nam* (which literally means South) refers to Vietnam and all things Vietnamese – a vernacular that reflects entangled identities beyond simple binaries. In a more recent development, during the 20th century, Vietnamese began to use three other terms to refer to traditional medicine: *Đông y* (Eastern medicine), *Y học cổ truyền* (traditional medicine), and *Y học dân tộc* (indigenous medicine). The conceptual rift between North and South – or China and Vietnam – were suddenly absorbed by the differentiation between the Vietnamese and the 'Western' or the 'modern' during this time. In practice, differences between Northern and Southern traditions of medicine still exist, however: Southern medicine uses few, if any, animal parts in its prescriptions, while Northern medicine invariably contains ingredients such as preserved snakes, dried insects, dried bats, and other bits and pieces of a variety of wildlife.

The turn to 20th-century neologisms also marks the institutionalization of non-biomedical therapeutic approaches in Vietnam: the word *học*, meaning studies, in *y học cổ truyền* and *y học dân tộc*, is hardly ever used outside of academic or institutional contexts to refer to Vietnamese medicine. Postcolonial institutions in Vietnam dedicated to non-biomedical scholarship and practice invariably adopt these neologisms in their names: *Viện Y học Cổ truyền* (Institute of Traditional Medicine), *Bệnh viện Y học Cổ truyền* (Traditional Medical Hospital), *Bệnh viện Y học Dân tộc* (Indigenous Medical Hospital), and *Viện Y Dược học Dân tộc* (Institute for the Study of Indigenous Pharmacy). *Hội Đông Y* (Association for Eastern Medicine) is an officially recognized, but not government-supported, organization; this, however, does not necessarily mean that *đông y* has the same negative connotation that 'Eastern medicine' usually does in languages such as Korean and Japanese (Thompson, 2015). The institutionalization of Vietnamese medicine in recent history is hardly unique; across South East Asia and among Asian superpowers such as China and India, various non-biomedical traditions have been enlisted in ongoing 'modernization' and 'scientization' projects that are closely tied to their postcolonial nation-building efforts (Scheid, 2002; Monnais et al., 2011; Lambert, 2018). Across East and South East Asia, practices of medical plurality (coexistence of multiple medical approaches), hybridization (active mixing of traditional and modern medicine), or synthesis (coming together of traditions) are the norm rather than a matter of deviation (Scheid, 2002; Rose, 2007). The body of non-biomedical knowledge that is codified and recognized by postcolonial governments is, however, nowhere near exhaustive: there exists what Lambert (2018) refers to as folk medicine, which exists alongside biomedicine and state-legitimated non-biomedical traditions, and is usually cast aside as quackery or harmless superstition.

In everyday conversation, Southern medicine and Northern medicine are used to refer to a range of non-biomedical therapeutic approaches and techniques that exist as living practices in Vietnam. These approaches coexist with their biomedical counterpart across all socioeconomic groups in different forms and to varying extents. Southern medicine is usually associated with empirical domestic medicine, where secret family recipes are usually shared for a fee, or passed along as gifts among friends (Monnais et al, 2011). Northern medicine is usually associated with a more learned and advanced tradition of the 'North' – in this case, referring to an ancient Sino-Vietnamese civilization that existed prior to Southern colonization of the Cham and the Khmer (modern central and Southern Vietnam) – which has a more comprehensive philosophy and sophisticated set of underlying theories (Marr, 1987). These common perceptions, however, largely overlooked the fact that 'miraculous' family recipes of Southern medicine were systematically documented and codified firstly by *Tuệ Tĩnh*, a 14th-century physician known as *Thánh thuốc Nam* (Saint of Southern medicine), and later on by *Hải Thượng Lãn Ông*, who was honoured as the Great Herb Doctor (*Đại Y Tông*), in the 18th century. In any case, this vernacular persists on the internet, where social media groups organize themselves around non-biomedical modalities such as Southern medicine and herbal medicine.

Elsewhere, Monnais and Tousignant (2006) and Marr (1987) noted that by and large, the majority of Vietnamese healers operated with little government hindrance and yet with even less assistance – a double oversight that allows them to 'practice free all over the country' without any form of institution. This is the case despite the fact that the administration of French Indochina actively introduced European scientific and medical ideas to Vietnam, and as part of their colonial logic of conquest, exercised strong disapproval of traditional Vietnamese medicine and its practitioners (Monnais, 2019). Furthermore, despite growing interest in Western scientific medicine in the 1920s and 1930s, as demonstrated by the publication of popular journals in Vietnamese *quốc ngữ*, French, and even Chinese during this period – Thompson (2015) observes that there was little corresponding denigration of traditional medicine in Vietnam – a development that stood in stark contrast with what happened with Chinese medicine in China in the same period. Monnais et al (2011) and Thompson (2015) attribute this development to both the nationalist push from below, common among many Asian countries in leading up to decolonization, and the continued need for medical care left unmet by the French colonial government from above, particularly in rural and remote areas. The authority of the traditional healer – sometimes also touted under the titles of 'miraculous doctors' (*thần y*) or 'doctors of good conscience' (*lương y*) – persists well into the digital age, with social media groups being built around traditional medical public figures who continue to 'practise free all over the country', and in many cases across the Vietnamese diaspora.

Miracle cures as vernacular tradition

The notion of the miracle cure in the Vietnamese context is historically tied not to appeals made by the faithful to the saints in the traditions of Islamic, Buddhist, Hindu, or Christian pilgrimage, but rather to the miraculous healing effects of the everyday garden and jungle herbs and plants. In this regard, the miracle cure in vernacular Vietnamese was first recorded in a systematic way by the 14th-century Buddhist monk *Tuệ Tĩnh*. In 1385, *Tuệ Tĩnh* was sent to China as part of a diplomatic party that included 20 Buddhist monks in a tribute mission to the Ming court. In the 14th-century East Asian diplomatic world, small countries routinely sent missions with presents or tributes to China to appease their great neighbour in the North; these missions often included people with special talents or skills, of which *Tuệ Tĩnh* was a prime example. A respected doctor and herbalist, he worked extensively with plants and was credited with having founded many medical gardens at several pagodas (Monnais et al, 2011). One of *Tuệ Tĩnh*'s major medical treatises, the *Nam Dược Thần Hiệu* 南 藥 神 效 [Miraculous Drugs of the South], was written while he lived in exile in China.

'Miraculous Drugs of the South' was designed to systematize the use of southern medicaments within the parameters of Chinese drug theory and to present 'southern' medicine to physicians at the Ming court; for this reason, *Tuệ Tĩnh* wrote in Chinese rather than in *Nôm*, the script which dominates his other works. *Tuệ Tĩnh* is believed to have sent copies of the *Nam Dược Thần Hiệu* back to Vietnam via a Vietnamese diplomatic mission, and copies of this work existed in the Vietnamese royal libraries prior to the Ming invasion in 1407 (Thompson, 2017a). Despite the involuntary nature of his travels, *Tuệ Tĩnh*'s journey to China and the medical text he produced during his time there had a significant impact on the development of Vietnamese traditional medical texts. That 'Miraculous Drugs of the South' was written in Chinese is often interpreted as *Tuệ Tĩnh*'s effort to elucidate Vietnamese medicine to his host country (Monnais et al, 2011; Thompson, 2015); the text itself appears to be a blend of a herbal handbook and a pragmatic guide, focusing on practical usage rather than theoretical aspects, to alleviate commonly encountered medical conditions.

Certain theoretical elements within the text, however, reveal an independent Vietnamese perspective on the natural world; a notable example of this can be seen in *Tuệ Tĩnh*'s approach to the *materia medica* section. Instead of adhering to Chinese classifications based on the Chinese Five Phases, he dives into presenting and categorizing the extraordinary drugs of his homeland based on their naturally occurring and easily observable physical similarities. Examples of these categories of miraculous drugs include: 'those derived from wild grasses and grass-like herbs', 'those derived from climbing plants', 'those derived from grasses that grow in water', 'those derived from grain-bearing plants', 'those derived from vegetables', 'those derived from rounded fruit and vegetables', 'those derived from trees', 'those derived from insects', 'those derived from animals with scales', 'those derived from fish', 'those derived from those with body armor/shells', 'those derived from those with shells', 'those derived from birds', 'those derived from water birds', 'those derived from domesticated animals', 'those derived from game animals', 'those from natural liquids', 'those from earth (dirt)', 'those derived from the five metals', 'those derived from stone', 'those derived from mineral salts', 'those derived from the human body', and so on. As far as is known, *Tuệ Tĩnh* was the only one to remain in China when the mission returned to *Đại Việt* – approximately the northern one third of the territory that comprises present-day Vietnam (Thompson, 2017a). That *Tuệ Tĩnh* was never allowed to return home and that his remains were never returned was a sore point with the people of *Tuệ Tĩnh*'s home village in *Cẩm Giàng, Hải Dương* province.

The miraculous cures of Vietnam, as such, reflect once again a long history of Northern imaginaries of the South. After a failed occupation of Vietnam (1407–27), Chinese rulers refrained from further attempts to include the region in the Chinese empire. Miasmic mist became an explanation for the political frontier or natural barrier of China (de Vries, 2022). The Chinese word for 'miasma' is etymologically related to the word 'barrier' (*zhang* 障). The 'miasmic climate' of Vietnam was understood as a 'deadly barrier' that set limits for military garrisons and Han settlements (Hanson, 2011, p 67). This understanding is consistent with the medical philosophy of *Tuệ Tĩnh*, which can be summarized as 'Vietnamese medicine for Vietnamese people' – in which a physical and spiritual relationship between Vietnamese people and the land where they live is foregrounded (Monnais et al, 2011). The effects of indigenous Vietnamese plants and herbs are miraculous in that they are explicitly understood to be contextually bound and culturally embodied. Even as they were systematized and became 'fixed' through the medium of the written word, in an important sense they do not travel very far.

The relationship between Vietnamese medicine, Vietnamese people, and Vietnam is understood to be inseparable: these are the conditions of possibility for Vietnamese miracle cures. Contrast this with faith healing, where people of faith go on long journeys of pilgrimage to sacred sites, shrines, or locations associated with miracles or revered religious figures to variously perform prayers, fasting, ablutions, and recitation of sacred texts, and participate in religious ceremonies in pursuit of miracle healing guidance, forgiveness, or direct intervention from a higher power. Sacred places are best understood as static containers of miracles; they lend themselves to various rituals of conjuring by the faithful whose connection with these places is conditioned by highly portable, highly mobile ideas about the self and its place in the world. The miracle cures of *Tuệ Tĩnh*, on the other hand, are almost stationary; they are bounded to his homeland, closed off onto itself, refusing to be readily codified.

Tuệ Tĩnh's writings assert that the earth, air, and water of the South produce foodstuffs and medicines which are uniquely suited to the Southern peoples he lived among; he maintained that good health is achieved by relying on seasonal local fruits and vegetables combined with a lifestyle of adequate physical exercise and moderation in hedonistic pursuits. Throughout his writings, *Tuệ Tĩnh* maintained that the botanical riches of Vietnam were superior for the Vietnamese people to imported Chinese medicines: a belief that corresponds with the historical exoticization of the non-Chinese of the Southern border, who routinely provided the antithesis in the defining of

Chineseness (Wade, 2000). The miraculous Other were often referred to in derogatory terms; terms such as *man*, *yi*, and *fan* were variously used to describe the people of the South who lacked the essential morality of human beings, whose characters were 'wily and deceitful', 'barbarous, rebellious and perverse' – portrayals in the Chinese historiographical tradition which has served to validate actions which the Chinese state took against such peoples (Wade, 2000, p 41). During its 20-year occupation of Vietnam, the Ming destroyed and confiscated Vietnamese books on diverse subjects such as medicine, history, and poetry and imported Chinese books carefully chosen for the schools the Chinese administrators had established (Hodgkin, 1981). The task of pacifying the South – codified in the name *An Nam* (Pacified South), a clipped form of the full name, the 'Protectorate General to Pacify the South' 安南都護府 (*An Nam đô hộ phủ*) – started in the year 679 under the Tang dynasty and continued well into the mid-20th century as various colonial powers came and went, even as Vietnam insisted on calling itself *Đại Cồ Việt* 大瞿越國 (968–1054), *Đại Việt* 大越國 [great Viet] (1054–1804), and ultimately *Việt Nam* under the *Nguyễn* dynasty (1804–1945). The miracle cures of the South, as it were, remained critical not only to the health of the Vietnamese population, but also to the Vietnamese project of national sovereignty.

Modern developments: institutionalization, internationalization, and regulation

Vietnam is a member state of the World Health Organization's (WHO's) Western Pacific Region Office (WPRO) – one of the six regions of the WHO. WPRO covers 37 countries and areas in Asia and the Pacific, with more than a quarter of the world's population (WHO, 2023). In 2012, WPRO published its regional *Traditional Medicine Strategy*, which provides guidelines for the development of national policies, regulations, and laws on traditional medicine (TM) among its member states. Vietnam is among the increasing number of countries and jurisdictions within WPRO implementing standards for Good Manufacturing Practices for herbal medicines and TM products. Vietnam has a national pharmacopoeia – among only nine WPRO countries with established national pharmacopoeias or monographs in 2010 (WHO, 2012). Neighbouring countries of the WHO's South-East Asia Regional Office (SEARO) also rallied under India's lead in adopting the *Delhi Declaration on Traditional Medicine* in February 2013, which saw 10 out of 11 countries in the region having national policies on TM in place. The push towards regulation and legitimization of non-biomedical knowledge and practices across Asia is emblematic of the professionalization and commercialization of practices outside of the mainstream biomedical enterprise.

Traditional medicine (*y dược cổ truyền*) in Vietnam is regulated by the Ministry of Health. According to Ministry of Health statistics, about 30 per cent of patients receive treatment with traditional medicine throughout Vietnam in a formal capacity. Although recent statistics are not available, it is recorded that there are about 1,000 traditional medicine practitioners, 5,000 traditional medical doctors, 2,000 assistant traditional medical doctors, and 209 traditional medicine pharmacists in 1998 (WHO, 2013). The Vietnam Association of Eastern Medicine Practitioners has over 70,000 members (Hoi Dong Y, 2019). Of this number, over 400 practitioners work in public hospitals (WHO, 2013). The Vietnam National Association of Acupuncture has over 27,000 members, 4,500 of whom work in public hospitals (Online Newspaper of the Government, 2012). There are 286 departments of traditional medicine in general hospitals, 45 provincial hospitals of traditional medicine, and four institutes of traditional medicine in Vietnam (WHO, 2013). The Vietnam Association of Southern Medicine [*Hội Nam Y Việt Nam*], established in 2016, had 2,250 members in 2021 and frequently published books and journals on Southern medicine, in addition to providing training to practitioners and organizing free medical examinations for the general public (Phu Nu Viet Nam, 2022). In 2022, the Vietnam Association of Southern Medicine changed its name to Vietnam Traditional Medicine Association [*Hội Y học Cổ Truyền Việt Nam*], consolidating various existing research, training, technologizing, publishing, and community outreach activities (Huong Thu, 2022).

There are three medical universities that have a faculty of traditional medicine, two pharmaceutical colleges, two secondary schools of traditional medicine, two state pharmaceutical companies, two state pharmaceutical manufacturers of herbal medicine, and three national research institutes for traditional medicine (WHO, 2013). There is a licensing system in place for traditional practitioners through an assessing committee: anyone who has 13 certificates issued by an assessing committee and the Ministry of Health can privately practise traditional medicine. The Ministry of Health also oversees The Vietnam Acupuncture Institute. The Institute is responsible for giving nationwide guidance on acupuncture and other medical therapies that reduce or avoid the use of drugs in treatment. The Institute hosts 350 beds and serves approximately 2,500 inpatients and 8,500 outpatients each year (WHO, 2013).

Article 39 of the Vietnamese Constitution outlines state undertakings to develop and integrate allopathic and traditional medical and pharmaceutical practices as well as to develop and integrate official health care, traditional medicine, and private medical care. 'Superstitious practice' is forbidden by Section 36 in the 1989 public health law. Before new treatment methods can be legally used, they must be approved by the Ministry of Health or provincial health office and the Traditional Medicine Association. Even though these measures are in place, there exists a large body of extralegal non-biomedical practices that are neither considered superstition nor officially recognized.

In their *Traditional Medicine Strategy 2014–2023* (extended to 2025), the WHO provided a roadmap designed to harness the potential contribution of traditional and complementary medicine (T&CM) to people-centred health care and promote therapeutically sound use of T&CM through regulation and national policies (WHO, 2013). Particularly, the strategy recommended the development of knowledge-based T&CM policies, where baseline data for the supervision of T&CM practices need to come from a comprehensive understanding of the specific nature of local T&CM sectors. Explicit questions need to be answered before a knowledge-based T&CM policy can be developed: why are people using T&CM, when are people using it, what are the benefits, who is delivering it, and what are their qualifications? Although these are fundamental questions, providing adequate answers often requires extensive resources that are not available to developing countries. In resource-poor contexts, economic constraints on data collection, monitoring, processing, dissemination, and publication are often worsened by poor institutional conditions and capacities that perpetuate non-standardization, non-structured information operations, and non-transparency. In the meantime, heavily subsidized internet access in these contexts has allowed people to perform increasingly significant parts of their everyday lives online as they generate a large amount of standardized and structured data.

In Vietnam and South East Asia, the issue of regulating non-biomedical practices is culturally and politically fraught (Monnais et al, 2011). Postcolonial governments across this region of newly independent states are eager to enlist traditional and indigenous medicines in various continuing 'modernization' and 'scientization' projects. These processes result in a body of state-legitimated non-biomedical practices that excludes a much larger uncodified yet popular set of practices, often regarded by the state as quackery or superstition (Wahlberg, 2007). As codified 'traditional' therapeutic approaches become incorporated into mainstream medical curricula, uncodified folk medicine proliferates through oral traditions, hand-me-down secret family recipes, and, most recently, via online social media networks on a much larger scale. Despite inherent tensions between the legitimate and the 'non-legitimate', these concurrent flows of knowledge and practices rally under the same banner of tradition as a means to create a sense of connection with the past through quasi-obligatory repetition of norms, values, and behaviours (Hobsbawm and Ranger, 2012). The invention or reconstruction of medical traditions as an activity that persists into modernity, therefore, is closely entwined with emerging cultural identities amid the changing state of global health inequities.

Miracle cures go digital: networks, inscriptions, and remediation

Miracle cures proliferate with a different temporality compared to scientific biomedicine; they ebb and flow through the totality of the highly structured, albeit pluralistic scientific enterprise. They rarely directly confront or challenge the logic of scientific knowledge; it is not in the interest of their survival to do so. As such, their temporality is also different from that of inaccurate understandings of scientific knowledge – the kind that would fuel conspiracy theories and eruptive events such as anti-vaccination movements. Inaccurate understandings of scientific knowledge and conspiracy theories are quick, short, reactive, and cyclical. The temporal currents of non-biomedical practices form new arms and channels as they branch out from the mainstream; new therapies and new interpretations of traditional texts are in constant negotiation with regulatory regimes, the traditions they build upon and veer off, and Science. What these new arms and channels lack in the authority that comes with established traditions, they make up for in their flexibility to adapt, hybridize, and reinvent themselves.

Digital expressions of miracle cures consolidate the oral, visual, and written forms that have historically mediated these healing practices. Social media, which are multimedia by design, create a space for these forms to coexist and interact in ways that were not previously possible. On Facebook, for example, people are enthusiastic in their advocacy of persistent drinking of papaya leaf tea to cure liver cancer, particular ways of massaging the face to cure haemorrhoids without the assistance of Western medicine, or blowing a hairdryer along one's spine and toes to cure COVID-19 symptoms. That these individual claims came to be understood as contingent miracle cures that could transcend subjectivities is a result of the intricate interplay between context, culture, and ongoing integration of digital technologies in everyday practices.

By situating the miracle cure in the context of technological mediation, we can begin to understand how miracle cures are taking on new hybrid analogue-digital forms. These hybrid forms could range from photos taken of hand-written miracle recipes to machine-readable inscriptions of miracle recipes as Facebook posts; from video-streamed tutorials of miracle cures to one-on-one miracle healing over livestreaming technologies. On one level, technology is enabling the digital codification of existing bodies of miracle cures through the migration of our dominant written culture onto social media. On a deeper level, it also affords opportunities for new miraculous healing practices to emerge with and through dynamic technologies such as video streaming and livestreaming, where the collapse of the oral and the visual over long distances and across temporalities fosters a sense of immediacy and communal participation, while allowing for the integration of speech and (machine and human) memory. Miracle cures as fluid, situational, and context-dependent modes of communication become an immediate and immersive experience by means of livestreaming technologies, where healing practices through mediated sensory stimulation follow a distinct logic of digital play, as we will explore in Part III.

Miracle cures as inscription networks

Network has become the predominant way with which we understand the internet and the information society. Since the turn of the century, research drawing on network techniques and concepts has proliferated across empirical domains and interests, and has become a mainstay in sociology, media studies, internet studies, and a range of other emergent disciplines. Network research in the past decade has shifted towards utilizing online interaction data generated as byproducts of everything we do on the internet to describe social processes through messy everyday interactions, experiment on network outcomes, and compare similar social processes across contexts. By way of inputting miraculous recipes in textual and visual formats, as well as commenting on, sharing, reposting, and appropriating these digital inscriptions, network actors leave behind traces that can be collected, assembled, analyzed, and made to speak.

Erikson (2013) observed that there are two distinct theoretical traditions to social network research: relationalism and formalism. Relationalism is a theoretical framework based on the primacy of relations rather than actor attributes; it rejects essentialism and *a priori* categories while emphasizing the intersubjectivity of experience and the content of interaction among actors, as well as their historical settings. Formalism, on the other hand, hails from the theoretical works of Georg Simmel,[1] which were preoccupied with identifying *a priori* categories of relational types and patterns that are independent of cultural content or historical settings. Any successful combination of the two approaches requires careful attention to the underlying presuppositions about perception, experience, and agency found in each. The formal social form focuses on patterns of ties at the expense of the content of those ties; this basic tenet has encouraged a body of research into network dynamics that completely (and deliberately) ignores the content of social ties. Social network research of the formalist flavour draws its analytical power from the ability to abstract away from details.

The fixity of formal social forms stands in contrast to the endless fluidity of a relationalist account of social life as open-ended, dynamic, and processual. For relationalists, meaning does not exist *a priori*, but rather emerges with and through interactions in co-constitutive ways. Erikson (2013) sharply remarks that another way of stating this approach would be to say that the meaning one individual assigns to another is the basis of any relationship; the absence of meaning can be interpreted as the absence of a relationship, in the sense that if one has no expectations or knowledge of another individual, then a relationship or connection cannot be said to exist. It is in this sense that meanings compose, rather than flow through, networks. Relationalism in sociology is usually positioned against substantialism – in which the source of social action and explanation in fixed entities exist independently of each other. These fixed entities can be individuals, societies, or social structures; when these fixed entities are said to interact, they are reified as if they were imbued with an existence of their own (Guy, 2018). The outcomes of these interactions exist in society, rather than constitute them. By contrast, concepts such as interaction, transaction, connection, and relation in the relationalist's arsenal of vocabulary call for a different way to think about social actors as mutually defining as they play their parts in a common process that unfolds over time – rather than disappear in it. Network analysis in the relational tradition does not aim to be transposable; it is meant to act as a useful analytical tool to make sense of particular settings. Indeed, network effects have been demonstrated to vary across contexts, providing a fruitful framework for researchers to conduct comparative studies in their relevant empirical domains.

This is not to say, however, that relational accounts of network do not make a claim on generalizability – or universality – but rather do so with and through context. Formalist generalizability is often devoid of context and culture, as formal social forms are understood as crystallized, locally defined structures of social relations that constrain individual behaviours and network outcomes (Erikson, 2013). As such, even though formalism and relationalism are logically inconsistent, they are internally consistent. Each has a commitment to generalizability that goes beyond the universalism vs. particularism dichotomy, and there are alternative approaches within these two traditions that hold the potential for working through their contradictions (Erikson, 2013). Frequently drawing on research from both approaches would enable researchers access to a large body of useful work across a wide variety of empirical domain. Erikson (2013) suggests that social network researchers could, apart from aligning themselves with one approach, also opt for professing theoretical pluralism (doing both), adopting a new theory powerful enough to encompass both approaches, and conducting empirical research exploring the areas of tension between the two research programmes.

Online social networks such as Facebook are built with a distinct logic of relational sociality. Facebook's description of itself reads: 'Facebook builds technologies that give people the power to connect with friends and family, find communities and grow businesses' (Facebook, 2021). The more connections one has on Facebook, the more depth there is to one's experience on this platform; it makes little sense for a frequent user to have a Facebook account (that is not a burner account – a social media account that one uses to post anonymously and avoid having their posts traced to them) with only a handful of connections. By extension, the more connections one has on these online networks, the more engaged and influential one is. To be in on the conversation in the context of online social networks is to follow platform logic – one that demands substantial user attention, which can be converted into data that help design more profitable platforms and sold to the rapidly increasing number of businesses that incorporate data-driven practices into their operations.

Behavioural data – the clicks, reacts, shares, comments, or group membership – are as important as the informational content being shared on these online social networks. Social media 'content' – a term reminiscent of the mass media era – comes in a variety of forms ranging from machine-readable texts, photos, and videos (pre-recorded or live stream). These units of content, constrained by platform affordances so that they can be automatically mined and retrieved for analysis post hoc, can be said to occupy their own network lives. However, these network lives are not detached from the social lives that precede and inform how they come about; indeed, they cannot be understood in separation from the underlying activities that have been digitized by virtue of people participating in these social networks. As much as digital behaviours are translations of social behaviours, social behaviours have also been reconfigured by the integration and augmentation of digital behaviours into everyday life.

In this entangled web of techno-social relationality, Actor–Network Theory (ANT) offers a promising invitation for *in situ* sense-making and sorting out relations and attachments. Despite its name, ANT is not so much a theory of network, but rather a theoretical movement[2] that instructs particular types of observation about how humans and non-humans assemble, come apart, and then come back together again – processes that resemble the formation and dissolution of networks. ANT views sociality not only on the level of association between humans and non-humans, but also from a dynamic of interaction between entities and categories, all of which produces problematic effects (Latour, 2005). ANT asks us to rethink the 'social' as bundles of ties that can be mobilized to account for some other phenomenon; it is only through following the 'actors' who interact with one another while leaving behind traces of network among themselves that the 'social' can properly be assembled. In other words, from a Latourian view, the social and network are one and the same: the social is never fixed, and there does not exist a social world outside of networks of relations among actors. This is what is meant by actor-networks: they are assemblages whose existence ceases as soon as the actors involved stop performing the interactions that characterize their relations.

While the instruction to 'follow the actor' neither explains nor outlines how this work is to be done, it suggests that the empirical field of work continuously emerges as a result of researcher engagement, and as such encouraging explorative and experimental ways of attuning to the world (Mol, 2008; Lury, 2021). ANT reminds us that particular modes of relating, though counter-intuitive to the existing ways in which we have come to understand human sociality in that they assert non-human agency, can open up the interconnected, consubstantial, co-constituted ways in which humans and non-humans mutually shape each other in and through their encounters. To this end, we can begin to assemble networks of the digital traces left behind by humans attempting to communicate with one another using social media platforms, using the same computational techniques that these platforms rely on for the ongoing maintenance of their infrastructure.

Computational techniques favour the written text over any other form of media: machine-readable text is by far the most computation-friendly communication format, lending itself to a plethora of automated data manipulation, measuring, and analysis (Tenen, 2017). This is a symptom of our writing society, which is saturated with traces and written objects (Lury, 2021). A significant portion of online space is textual space; the procedures that enable digital inscriptions, as formalized and standardized as they may be, are always in the process of update, validation, and control. The forms and materiality of texts are also active, fully-fledged elements of meaning themselves, which cannot be detached from written artefacts (Lury, 2021). In assembling the sociality of network operations, it seems, the written text offers a good starting point for the study of the simultaneous becoming of both the ordering technology of writing and the fragile, messy practices of creating and circulating digital inscriptions. Following this approach, Chapter 3 approaches scientific publications as literary inscriptions and presents a co-word analysis of the disparate literatures on traditional medicine, herbal medicine, alternative and complementary medicine, unorthodox cures, and unconventional medicine to reconceptualize miracle cures as non-biomedical knowledge.

Remedy remediation: the hypermediacy of digital cures

Formal analyses of behavioural textual data (such as the kind done in Part II) tells only part of the story. The lived experiences of people who rely on miracle cures for their survival – be it in their professional practice of these modalities as a primary mode of income, or in their engagement with these modalities as a tactic of managing the experiences of illness of their own and their loved ones – cannot be captured through formal analysis. The activities and stories that leave no discernible trace on social media platforms, and yet happen alongside these traces, are an integral part of the story. These events are as much a part of the technologies as the traces themselves; for this reason, we can say that the suite of media technologies embedded on social media are agents in our culture without falling into the trap of technological determinism. Digital technologies, such as livestreaming and videostreaming, are not external agents that come to disrupt an unsuspecting culture; rather, they emerge from within cultural contexts and refashion other media that came before them, as well as those which are embedded in similar contexts. A recipe shared as text on Facebook has a different malleability and tractability to a video instructing viewers on how to follow the same recipe – or to suggestions on where to buy the necessary ingredients, or philanthropic offers to mail ingredients to those who want them. At the same time, dynamic practices such as livestreaming miracle cures or performing miracle cures through livestreaming are reconfiguring what it means to enact these miracles. Introducing digital technologies into miracle cure practices does not simply entail acquiring new hardware and mastering the use of software; rather, digital cures entail the fashioning and refashioning of existing material, social, aesthetic, and economic assemblages of practice.

Tracing the theory of remediation as the oscillation between the logics of immediacy and hypermediacy, Bolter and Grusin (1999) argued that new and emerging media refashion prior media forms so that the presence of the previous media cannot be totally effaced. Rather than transcending earlier media forms, new media variously comment on, reproduce, and replace media forms that coexist within a particular media ecology; these remediations are capable of reforming realities through the insertion of their own agential functioning, whose actions are never divorced from the specific contexts in which they operate. Immediacy refers to the manner in which a media provides a window through to the live event, while hypermediacy refers to the heightened awareness of the different windows used to achieve the mediated experience among media participants. For Bolter and Grusin (1999), although each medium promises to reform its predecessors by offering a more immediate or authentic experience, the promise of reform inevitably leads us to become aware of the new medium as a medium – hence the oscillation between mediacy and hypermediacy (and also transparency and opacity). In the proliferation of multiplying media, the presence of media is continually made apparent (hypermediacy); this is the case despite efforts to smooth over the mediated experience in service of authenticity (immediacy). As such, neither total immediacy nor total hypermediacy is possible or desirable; by borrowing or repurposing from an earlier medium, new media refashion not only the content (for example, digitized textual miracle recipes), but also the medium (for example, performing transnational miracles through livestreaming technologies).

Throughout the book, as we explore the social lives of digital miracles from Vietnam, we also explore the universality in the media forms that they have taken on – as well as the contingent performances of miracle cures with and through technology. Social media platforms remediate various forms of communication while implementing automated means of curating, moderating, and regulating both social media content and its forms. These dynamic and changing processes condition and co-evolve alongside mediated practices, including that of miracle healing and the digital propagation of miracle recipes. In the next chapter, we will further position miracle cures as practices that persist alongside the pluralistic practices of biomedicine by examining a large dataset of more than 30 years' worth of scholarly literature across different disciplines.

3

Miracle Cures as
Non-Biomedical Practices

The naming of things matters. What we decide to call a thing, however arbitrarily, does not merely provide us with a convenient point of reference for that thing; the act of naming enlists the empirical subject in a web of meanings that both precedes it and is produced by it. Calling a range of therapeutic modalities 'complementary' and 'alternative' has the effect of clarifying and solidifying what it means to be 'scientific', while at the same time alienating and marginalizing what lies outside of this scientific framework. Once a naming convention has become stabilized, the semantic network built around this name is anything but arbitrary. Once we have decided that a medicine is 'unorthodox' or 'traditional', for example, it is less straightforward to associate it with things like 'rigour', 'efficacy', or 'government funding'. Names represent the empirical object as they designate general qualities and substances that sustain the possibility of discourse about that object; it is through this discursivity of language that the construction of knowledge becomes possible. Names as signifiers, similar to all of language, are not always perfect; their imperfections and errors, however, record what has been learned and allow for the progression of knowledge through judgement of what is being proposed, articulated, and derived from naming conventions.

Some naming activities are more formal and formalized than others. The naming of specialties within scientific medicine, for example, has grown increasingly systematic and narrowly focused. The General Medical Council (GMC) in the UK records more than 65 specialties and 31 sub-specialties in formal biomedical pedagogy; the Association of American Medical Colleges (AAMC) records more than 160 specialties and subspecialties, while the Medical Board of Australia (MBA) recognizes over 80 scientific medical specialties and fields of specialty practice (MBA, 2018; AAMC, 2023; GMC, 2023). The naming of specialities inevitably informs practice; by the mid-1950s, medical specialization had become a fundamental characteristic of biomedicine (Weisz, 2006). At the same time, the naming of non-Western, non-scientific therapeutic modalities in scholarly literature proliferates in a much less systematic manner. This contrast is not incidental; it is the result of a structural reordering of medical epistemology at the dawn of clinical sciences.

Using a network approach, this chapter analyzes the naming conventions in scholarly knowledge produced about the therapeutic knowledge and practices that precede and persist alongside biomedical knowledge. This network approach takes the proliferation of naming activities in scholarly knowledge production as a productive site of interrogation. More specifically, it takes these names as *literary inscriptions* around which problematic networks of knowledge production are constructed. The chapter begins by historicizing the institutionalization of biomedicine and its impact on miracle cures as non-biomedical: that is, as modalities that have been displaced and marginalized by the scientific enterprise. It proceeds by articulating the theoretical approach that conceptualizes knowledge production as problematic networks, before reviewing the proliferation of terms used to denote the non-biomedical in English-language scholarly literature. The chapter then presents an original co-word analysis of disparate literatures on non-biomedical modalities from 1980 to 2022, which maps the overlapping knowledge domains that exist within a contemporaneous scholarly corpus on the topic. From this analysis, I refine my conceptualization of miracle cures as non-biomedical modalities while advancing the argument that we should understand therapeutic modalities that exist at the margin of scientific medicine in historical relation to the biomedical. I argue that we should contend with the historical disruption that biomedicine both as a scientific discipline and as a mechanism of body surveillance came to solidify modernity around the world precisely by highlighting this disruption in the way we talk about the non-biomedical. As we saw in Chapter 2, Vietnamese miracle cures continue to persist well into the scientific age through continuing modernization and scientization. A historically informed approach to conceptualizing miracle cures across context is needed.

The birth of biomedicine and the marginalization of non-biomedical modalities

In the 1963 book *The Birth of the Clinic*, Foucault characterized a critical 'turning point' in the history of 18th-century Western medicine that came with the institution of the *clinique*, in which the medical gaze created an epistemic break between medical knowledge and non-knowledge. The advent of the clinical science of medicine is part and parcel of a wider reorganization of the structure of knowledge that champions empiricism, which subsequently shapes what gets included in medical discourse and constrains the very possibility of discourse about disease. The 18th-century medical gaze did not simply direct itself towards the human body in a more refined manner as a result of accumulated scientific progression. Between the Morgagnian gaze towards the sick body as a local host of organ-level diseases and the Bichatian gaze towards pathological tissues and membranes is an epistemic rupture that stabilized the body as a site for temporal readings of disease, argued Foucault.

The stethoscope as an early 19th-century medical technology further endowed this medical gaze with a 'plurisensorial' structure that renders the body invisible visible, transforming the medical gaze into a totality that designates anything outside its purview as beyond the domain of knowledge. Medical technologies have since grown increasingly sophisticated; the panoptic surveillance of the human body has evolved to include the X-ray machine, MRIs, CT scans, DXA scans, sonograms, and emerging 3D interactive visualization techniques. Sophisticated medical imaging techniques are only part of a wide array of modern biomedical technologies, however. Lock and Nguyen (2010), for example, remind us that biomedical sciences are actively constructed by biomedical technologies, which straddle sociotechnical institutions such as hospitals, laboratories, biotech companies, and the state. The mundane, everyday biomedical technologies that pervade modernity also include techniques and activities ranging from basic physical examination and patient history-taking to administration of injection and prescription of medication. Biomedicine exercises an authoritative control over the human body as it displaces and marginalizes non-biomedical practices (Lock and Nguyen, 2010). This subjugation, however, is neither linear nor comprehensive; non-biomedical knowledge and practices continue to exist across the world, and the interaction between the biomedical and the non-biomedical continues to evolve in both clinical and non-clinical settings (Shorofi and Arbon, 2017; Tovey et al, 2017; Lindquist et al, 2018).

This chapter seeks to define non-biomedical knowledge and practices as therapeutic modalities that exist in separation, but not isolation from, biomedicine. This separation is multiple. There is an ongoing epistemological separation, with non-biomedical knowledge usually lacking epistemic 'virtues' such as precision, certainty, and replicability. At the same time, biomedical knowledge lacks certain aspects of the ontologies that support the epistemologies of various non-biomedical practices. This separation is also historical (with biomedical knowledge inextricably linked to modernity and modernization), social (access and subscription to non-biomedical regimens are socially stratified and stratifying), cultural (with biomedical knowledge supposedly freed from value and emotion, allowing it to be wholesale transported across cultures), and institutional (with the professionalization of biomedicine consolidating its credentials and market opportunities while excluding non-biomedical practices).

Partly existing outside the formal and highly regulated health sector, non-biomedical therapeutic practices persist as living cultures that also often incorporate biomedical technologies and techniques. Examples of these hybrid practices include X-ray scanning use among chiropractors (Ernst, 1998), eclectic combining use of Viagra and traditional Chinese medicine among men being treated for impotence (Zhang, 2007), use of traditional medicine among cancer patients in India (Broom et al, 2009), and agnostic evaluation of blood test results in conjunction with Eastern medical diagnosis among Vietnamese women being treated for infertility (Pashigian, 2012). In other cases, hybridity is negotiated and less straightforward. An example of this is the case of the *haad vaidya* (bone doctors) in India, where, despite these doctors' assertion of manual diagnosis as their core competence, patients bring along X-ray scans to consultation on their own initiative (Lambert, 2012). Living practices of non-biomedical therapies are guided by an acute pragmatism that allows both non-biomedical practitioners and their patients to navigate a highly complex landscape of medical pluralism. This navigation allows patients to negotiate individualized treatments that reflect culturally and politically conditioned understandings and circumstances of health and illness. As such, non-biomedical modalities are practices that managed to escape the totality of the 20th-century biomedical gaze only insofar as they partially reject, and are rejected by, scientifically circumscribed sites of biomedical knowledge.

Knowledge production as problematic networks

Since the mid-19th century, doctors increasingly rely on laboratory sciences to inform their practice (Löwy, 2011). Post-World War II marks a period of 'biomedicalization', wherein biomedicine as a term coined during the interwar period is used as a shorthand for the intermingled practices of doctors and scientists (Löwy, 2011). Even though the processes of biomedicalization are heterogeneous – some medical disciplines were faster than others in turning to the laboratory – increasingly dense networks of doctors, scientists, and industrialists were mobilized as a result of health-care funding, government regulation, and patient activism (Bell and Figert, 2015).

The centrality of the laboratory as a locus that exercises power over the shaping of development and the transformation of post-industrial society is recognized in sociological writings (Touraine, 1971, 1977; Latour, 1993). Displacing the industrial firm in the same way that the industrial firm downgraded the state, and in the same way that the state displaced religious organizations that came before, knowledge organizations such as laboratories, hospitals, and research centres are what Touraine (1971) considers to be the strategic loci of social change. The production of knowledge within these knowledge organizations is always politically charged; it is not possible to lean on the 'ivory tower' model and paint an accurate picture of scientific innovation (Latour, 1988, 1993).

Scientific knowledge production, therefore, does not happen within 'specialist communities' who carve out 'research areas' that are independently defined and delimited (Latour and Woolgar, 1979; Callon et al, 1986; Latour, 1988). Knowledge production in the sciences is better described as problematic socio-cognitive networks of hybrid communities, whose interests are aggregated and funnelled through *translations* of scientific publications as *literary inscriptions* (Callon et al, 1983). In this translation process, all actors involved build around them complex and changing networks of elements that are linked together and made dependent upon the actors themselves. These actors are heterogeneous in nature; they can be individuals, organizations, or concepts. Translation as well as counter-translation of and by these actors make network associations possible; they constitute a language better equipped to identify knowledge production in multidisciplinary and transdisciplinary research than the Kuhnian 'paradigms' of highly focused scientific disciplines, or the Mertonian 'clusters' of scientific authority. Within this framework, words as they are positioned and stabilized within literary inscriptions act as *translation operators* (Callon et al, 1983) that allow actors to navigate and consolidate webs of interests. Translation operators, identified and extracted from their inscriptions and subsequently reassembled without relying on pre-established classification schemes, can reveal poles of interest, their convergence or intersection, relationships that are developed around them, and the general configuration of the problematic network (Callon et al, 1983).

As the next section will show, understanding knowledge production as problematic networks is particularly useful to the task of uncovering the knowledge structure of English-language scholarly literature on non-biomedical modalities. Scholarly knowledge about non-biomedical modalities is organized in neither definitive paradigms nor stable and discrete clusters: this is evidenced in the absence of terminology consensus and established authority across disciplinary inquiries. In a sense, production of scholarly knowledge about knowledge that escapes the totality of the scientific gaze seems to reflect what Daston and Galison (2007) refer to as the plurality of 'visions of knowledge'. This plurality of visions will remain a permanent feature of the scientific enterprise due to its capacious commitment to fidelity to 'nature' – in this case, the therapeutic modalities that exist outside of the highly ordered scientific way of knowing. The proliferation of problematic terminologies used to describe non-biomedical modalities in literature is an example of such a commitment. This commitment, however, could be detrimental to its subject if these plural visions of knowledge impose partial and politically fraught views of what constitutes the subject of scientific inquiry (Daston and Galison, 2007).

Contested terminologies on non-biomedical modalities: a literature review

Since the turn of the millennium, a number of attempts have been made to categorize the various concepts surrounding non-biomedical therapeutic modalities, although none has been exhaustive or conclusive. Nigenda et al (2001), for example, developed a heuristic scheme of three non-biomedical categories based on their survey on medical pluralism in Morelos, Mexico, comprising traditional medicine, alternative medicine, and faith healing. However, this heuristic scheme is highly specific to the context of Mexican medical pluralism and cannot be generalized. For example, traditional medicine is defined within this typology as 'the outcome of the syncretic union between pre-Hispanic concepts and health care practices' (p 12), whereas alternative medicine is defined as 'a wide variety of concepts and practices which have distinct and non-indigenous origins, ranging from Chinese acupuncture to European homeopathy' (p 12). Nigenda et al (2001) also mentioned a range of terminologies from existing literature that are neither clearly defined nor sufficiently analyzed, such as herbal medicine, indigenous medicine, complementary medicine, unconventional medicine, unorthodox medicine, and religious healing – which are conceptualized in opposition to 'technologized medicine' and 'pharmaceutical medicine'. The ease with which terminologies seem to proliferate in this domain is indicative of a lack of consensus and an absence of established disciplinary authority. This proliferation also suggests a diverse range of perspectives from which non-biomedical modalities become interesting to scholarly research. The semantic plurality that results from these perspectives does not signify a lack of precision or engagement; it is suggestive of the overlapping conceptual spaces that might lay dormant in the literature.

A close look at published papers citing Nigenda et al (2001) yields an even more diverse set of vocabularies, including natural medicine, national medicine, popular medicine, ethnomedicine, ethnobotany, plant-based medicine, and integrative medicine. These terms are conceptualized against 'dominant medicine' and 'modern medicine' (Napolitano and Mora Flores, 2003; Han and Ballis, 2007; Waldstein, 2010; Gale, 2014; Olson, 2016). Waldstein (2010) also mentioned *materia medica* as the European codification of medicinal plants both introduced and native to the context of Mexico. There also seems to be dissatisfaction among researchers with existing terminologies; this is largely due to the ideological undertone that informs much of research about the marginalized non-scientific. Reflecting on the evolving status of non-biomedical modalities in the United States, Cassidy (2008) demonstrates how non-biomedical modalities evolved from being referred to as 'unorthodox' in the first Chantilly Conference organized by the National Health Institute in 1992 to subsequent labels of 'alternative', 'complementary' (adapted from the European *Komplementarmedizin*), and, most recently, 'integrative'. What remains unchanged in this decade-long evolution of terminologies in the US, argued Cassidy (2008), is the latent 'Us vs Them' dichotomy which fails to recognize a moral economy that regulates this discourse in favour of the ontological privilege of biomedicine. Furthermore, Murphy et al (2003) illustrate that optimal retrieval of literature on complementary and alternative medicine is highly difficult due to inconsistent thesaurus use among popular databases. This inconsistency is partly attributable to the fact that terms used to denote non-biomedical modalities are defined differently across different countries and even among different research groups within the same country (Wootton, 2005).

The proliferation of terms in this domain is also reflective of the highly insular discourse that happens on a disciplinary level. Kaptchuk and Eisenberg (2001), for example, developed a taxonomy of what they called 'unconventional healing practices'. This taxanomy contains two main taxa, namely complementary and alternative medicine (CAM) and parochial unconventional medicine. They explicitly built this taxonomy based on the level of appeal ascribed to different therapeutic modalities, determined by the size of their subscription base. Based on these criteria, non-biomedical modalities can either appeal to the general public (CAM) or to specific ethnic or religious groups (parochial unconventional medicine). Despite drawing on a diverse set of therapeutic approaches, Kaptchuk and Eisenberg's taxonomy is constructed from a biomedicine-centric worldview and is heavily motivated by the logic of 'taming' patient behaviour. The taxonomy was developed primarily as a guide for physicians to understand patients' reactions to illness and assist them in ensuring compliance. A taxonomy of this kind is not without its own disciplinary merit; what it fails to recognize, however, is the politics of the subject matter at hand. Bates (2000), for example, pointed out that it makes just as much sense to call biomedicine or modern medicine 'alternative medicine', given its unique position in history and culture as a therapeutic approach. Recognizing the fact that a historical anomaly came to be understood as the 'standard' against which all other past and present medical practices are measured does not diminish its worth. Clarifying the historical ontology of biomedicine can help uncover the hegemonic processes that marginalize the medicines which escaped the 'biomedical turn', while problematizing the modernist fallacy that fails to explain the continuing persistence and popularity of non-biomedical practices.

Elsewhere, Caspi et al (2003) call for a turn to the patient to combat 'societal mega-stereotypes' that permeate the confusions surrounding definitions of CAM. Arguing that it is fallacious to lump hundreds of heterogeneous therapeutic modalities under the same label, Caspi et al (2003) point out inconsistencies in what constitutes CAM across different

US national statistics organizations, among doctors with university versus private hospital affiliations, and among laypeople versus experts. Echoing the call to recognize diversity while being precise about the nuances of various medicines' ongoing trajectories, Cassidy (2008) recommends paying attention to specialization trends within non-biomedical practices, minding the differences in scale that separate modalities from therapies, and referring to specific modalities by their names. Most of these individual names are indicative of the therapeutic cultures in which they are embedded (*Ayurveda, Unani, curanderismo*) and their geo-political identities (Traditional Chinese medicine, Southern Vietnamese medicine, Tibetan medicines). This call for viewing non-biomedical modalities as 'things in themselves' highlights the significance of semantics in this domain. The naming and classification of practices are value-ridden activities; their semantic shifts create opportunities for new beneficiaries of these interpretations to emerge.

More than a decade has passed since Cassidy's (2008) recommendations on streamlining terminology use were proposed, yet the landscape of scholarly discourse about non-biomedical modalities remains conceptually ambiguous. Templeman, Robinson and McKenna (2015) conducted a study into medical students' conceptualization of 'complementary medicine' and 'complementary and alternative medicine' within their discourse community only to find that what these terms mean varies depending on context, and once again called for a revisit of terminology use. Concluding that terminology use for complementary medicine is not definitive and that there might never be universal agreement on the meanings of different terms used to describe non-biomedical modalities, they predict, however, that a progression towards the term 'integrative medicine' is inevitable in order to facilitate legitimacy and acceptance of complementary medicines by the medical community (Templeman et al, 2015). However, it remains unclear whether this supposedly inclusive term will be embraced by the scholarly community, how long it will take for this to happen, and what implications this semantic shift will have on knowledge in this area. The discourse of integration is not without problem; it remains elusive what should be integrated, how this integration should take place, whether the integration has indeed happened, and who should decide the course of this integration.

Finding a way forward: a co-word analysis of literature

Our discussion so far has demonstrated a multiplicity of terms that permeates the articulation of non-biomedical modalities in scholarly literature. This multiplicity is fundamentally different from the systematic growth in vocabulary that orders the language of biomedical literature. Foucault (1966) distinguishes between horizontal and vertical articulation in the general grammar of naming. The naming of scientific biomedicine is being articulated horizontally: this is achieved both through the grouping together of common individual specialties and modalities and their sequential generalization, as well as through the infinite subdivision of these groups into evolving distinctions. The articulation of non-biomedical modalities and specialties, on the other hand, is vertical: it is through descriptions of modifications, features, accidents, and characteristics that naming proliferates within this domain. This articulation is formularized through the predominant 'adjective + medicine' convention that seems to have been taken for granted. While horizontal articulation lends itself to taxonomy and nomenclature through increasing generalities and specificities, vertical articulation is substantive: it creates names that subsist by themselves in discourse. Structuring and ordering the vertical articulation of non-biomedical modalities are not straightforward tasks; they are important tasks nevertheless, as a discourse overburdened by a multiplicity of terms is also one susceptible to confusion.

A more systematic approach to analyzing the conceptual landscape of literatures on non-biomedical terminologies would refresh our approach. In a space where universal consensus seems unattainable and terminology proliferation is the norm, it is useful to map out how these terminologies and their associated conceptual networks emerge and relate to one another using quantitative methods. By visualizing the problematic socio-cognitive networks of these contested terminologies, dormant domains of meaning and conceptual spaces can be excavated and brought to life. This mapping exercise also helps substantiate and clarify the separation that exists between biomedicine and non-biomedicine within scholarly literature: the degrees of their separation, their boundaries, features within their territories, and any bridges that link them together.

A systematic mapping exercise of this nature requires systematic literature retrieval. Our thematic discussion so far has provided us with 18 common terminologies used in literature. These terminologies are alternative medicine, traditional medicine, herbal medicine, complementary medicine, *materia medica*, integrative medicine, ethnobotany, ethnomedicine, natural medicine, faith healing, popular medicine, indigenous medicine, national medicine, plant-based medicine, religious healing, unconventional medicine, nonbiomedical modalities, and unorthodox medicine. These terms relate to one another on a systemic level: they are referred to either in the same document, or in documents citing one another. These terms therefore could be used as search terms for a systematic retrieval of literature. The corpus generated from this systematic retrieval can in turn be analyzed quantitatively, allowing us to operationalize discursive structures underpinning the production of knowledge in this field.

This chapter presents a systematic mapping of the extant literatures referencing non-biomedical therapeutic modalities by adopting a network approach. A structured search of document keywords, titles, and abstracts from 1980 to 2022 was conducted on Scopus using 18 search terms. Scopus is the largest citation and abstract database of peer-reviewed literature. The strings entered for this search are 'alternative medicine', 'traditional medicine', 'herbal medicine', 'complementary medicine', 'materia medica', 'integrative medicine', 'ethnomedicine', 'natural medicine', 'faith healing', 'popular medicine', 'indigenous medicine', 'national medicine', 'plant-based medicine', 'religious healing', 'unconventional medicine', 'nonbiomedical⋆', and 'unorthodox medicine'. It is estimated that Scopus covers around 87 million records of literature spanning the life sciences, social sciences, physical sciences, and health sciences (Elsevier, 2023).

From the structured search, a dataset of 33,699 bibliographic records was generated. The dataset was retrieved on 7 July 2023. These records represent the contemporaneous scientific corpus produced by the most recent generation of researchers over the past 30+ years. The dataset contains the following elements: author name, author affiliation, publication title, year of publication, journal title, abstract, keywords provided by publication authors, keywords indexed by Scopus, and citation count. Only the most-cited 20,000 records for each search term were exported due to restrictions imposed by Scopus. There are three search terms that returned more than 20,000 records. Table 3.1 provides an overview of the dataset. This corpus is made up of the most cited scientific publications in the field that is commonly known as traditional, complementary, and alternative medicine (TM/CAM). A variety of bibliometric analyses can be conducted on such a dataset, including word frequency analysis, citation analysis, co-word analysis, simple document counting (Thelwall, 2008), and semantic title-abstract-keyword content analysis (Meyer and Schroeder, 2009).

I conducted a co-word analysis (Callon et al, 1983, 1986, 1991) on the keywords collected from the dataset. Co-word analysis, whose theoretical roots trace back to Actor-Network Theory, is a method widely used in bibliometric and scientometric studies (He, 1999; Börner et al, 2003; Yang et al, 2012; Igami et al, 2014). Co-word analysis was developed partly in response to the limitations of co-citation analysis, which tends to overemphasize highly focused 'specialty areas' in scientific research where knowledge transformations are sudden and radical (Callon et al, 1983). Co-word analysis has been used for a variety of research purposes, including knowledge discovery (He, 1999; Ronda-Pupo and Guerras-Martin, 2012; Lv et al, 2018), hypothesis generation (Stegmann and Grohmann, 2003), and mapping intellectual structures of scientific disciplines (Ravikumar et al, 2015; Flis and van Eck, 2018; Corrales-Garay et al, 2019). Co-word analysis is an effective quantitative method to account for the heterogeneity of actors and concepts involved in problematic networks of knowledge. In carrying out co-word analysis, we can identify certain patterns of clustering among and between the scientific papers recorded in the current corpus; by subsequently performing a semantic content analysis, we can see which thematics appear as prevalent in each of these clusters. Within the corpus, certain forms of clustering around particularly dominant keywords can be observed; within those clusters, we can also observe some semantic affinities (see Figure 3.1).

There are two types of keywords in this dataset: keywords provided by publication authors (author keywords), and keywords provided by Scopus (index keywords, or subject headings). Scopus assigns subject headings to both individual publications and the journals in which they are published (Elsevier, 2023). Scopus claims to manually index 80 per cent of the publications it stores, using seven separate controlled vocabularies/thesauri (Elsevier, 2023). Inclusion of all subject headings provides an added layer of translation imposed upon relevant modalities, which is suitable to the purpose at hand. Indexing as a socio-cognitive practice does not generally aim at summarizing document content; the objective is to identify interests relevant to different specialists (Callon et al, 1983; 1991). Both types of keywords therefore act as active translation operators that define conceptual domains while establishing their relationships with a series of other domains. As a result, networks constructed from these translation operators provide a map of inscriptions, and a map of chosen inscriptions in turn provides an insight into the ontologies so inscribed. These ontologies are important in the construction of the socio-cognitive foundations of diverse scientific communities.

Co-word analysis of 890 keywords which co-occurred at least 80 times across 33,699 bibliographic entries results in four conceptual clusters, as shown in Figure 3.1. While depth is lost when working with such a large dataset, there are gains in terms of mapping the topography and patterns of publication in this field. The semantic topography produced as a result of this co-word analysis (Figure 3.1) was generated using VOSViewer (van Eck and Waltman, 2009a; 2017). VOSViewer is an application widely used in scientometrics. VOSViewer generates two-dimensional maps by combining two techniques: mapping and clustering. The mapping technique employed in this program is called VOS, which is closely related to multidimensional scaling (van Eck et al, 2010). The clustering technique employed in this program is closely related to modularity-based clustering (Waltman et al, 2010; van Eck and Waltman, 2017). The result is a map that illustrates the relatedness of keywords as translation operators in two dimensions: distance (mapping) and colour (clustering). Keywords that share the same colour (belonging to the same cluster) appear more frequently together than keywords that have a different colour. The distance between keywords is constructed based on the software's built-in attraction and repulsion parameters; the closer two keywords are on the map, the more closely related they are to each other.

Semantic topography of literature

An overview of the dataset is presented in Table 3.1, sorted by number of results. From the table, we can see that traditional medicine, alternative medicine, and herbal medicine are the most used terms in the literature. Additionally, they share the same most cited paper; this paper is also the most cited paper in the dataset. This triple popularity signals the dominant narrative in scholarly discourse on non-biomedical therapeutic modalities. This narrative presents non-biomedical modalities in ideological terms ('alternative' – circumscribing an undefined 'otherness'), against teleological scientific progress ('traditional' – reminiscing of a pre-modern cultural past), and against systematic scientific experimentation ('herbal' – evoking a kind of crudeness that diametrically opposes synthetic pharmaceutical biomedicine).

The next rows in Table 3.1, namely ethnobotany, complementary medicine, integrative medicine, and *materia medica*, return significantly fewer records. These terms signal the 'scientization' of non-biomedical modalities that are common to both Western and non-Western contexts. This 'scientization' is manifested through acknowledging uses of natural resources prior to the advent of science ('materia medica'), while giving them legitimacy only within the confinement of scientific medical discourse ('complementary' and 'integrative').

Figure 3.1 presents the semantic topography of non-biomedical modalities as a result of co-word analysis. The weight of each concept – visualized by the size of each corresponding node – represents its total link strength. Total link strength is defined as the sum of the number of links a node shares with all other nodes in the network. Clusters are determined by the association strength method (van Eck and Waltman, 2009b), a probabilistic measure which normalizes co-occurrence data to calculate direct similarity. Concepts that belong to the same cluster are represented in the same colour; they co-occur more frequently than those outside their cluster. The most densely populated cluster is marked in red (344 nodes), followed by green (275 nodes), blue (149 nodes), and finally yellow (122 nodes). These clusters are numbered from 1 to 4, respectively. Not all nodes are visible in Figure 3.1 due to the limits of two-dimensional visualization.

Concepts with the highest number of links are considered the most central/influential within their respective clusters. These nodal modalities are: alternative medicine (cluster 1), unclassified drug (cluster 2), herbal medicine (cluster 3), and traditional medicine (cluster 4). 'Unclassified drug' was not included in the original search strings; however, our analysis indicates that it is one of the most used terms in literature. For our purpose,

Table 3.1: Overview of results

Strings entered	Results	Most cited paper	Citations
'Traditional medicine'	55,608	Trends in alternative medicine use in the United States, 1990–1997: Results of a follow-up national survey. Eisenberg, D.M., Davis, R.B., Ettner, S.L., (...), Van Rompay, M., Kessler, R.C. 1998 *Journal of the American Medical Association* 280(18), pp 1569–75	6,040
'Alternative medicine'	53,129	Trends in alternative medicine use in the United States, 1990–1997: Results of a follow-up national survey. Eisenberg, D.M., Davis, R.B., Ettner, S.L., (...), Van Rompay, M., Kessler, R.C. 1998 *Journal of the American Medical Association* 280(18), pp 1569–75	6,040
'Herbal medicine'	47,766	Trends in alternative medicine use in the United States, 1990–1997: Results of a follow-up national survey. Eisenberg, D.M., Davis, R.B., Ettner, S.L., (...), Van Rompay, M., Kessler, R.C. 1998 *Journal of the American Medical Association* 280(18), pp 1569–75	6,040
'Ethnobotany'	8,020	Medicinal plants: Traditions of yesterday and drugs of tomorrow. Gurib-Fakim, A. 2006 *Molecular Aspects of Medicine* 27(1), pp 1–93	1,310
'Complementary medicine'	7,551	Use of complementary and alternative medicine in cancer patients: A European survey. Molassiotis, A., Fernandez-Ortega, P., Pud, D., (...), Kearney, N., Patiraki, E. 2005 *Annals of Oncology* 16(4), pp 655–63	830
'Integrative medicine'	6,250	Effectiveness of acupuncture as adjunctive therapy in osteoarthritis of the knee. A randomized, controlled trial. Berman, B.M., Lao, L., Langenberg, P., (...), Gilpin, A.M.K., Hochberg, M.C. 2004 *Annals of Internal Medicine* 141(12), pp 901–10+I-20	503
'Materia medica'	5,101	Historical Perspective of Traditional Indigenous Medical Practices: The Current Renaissance and Conservation of Herbal Resources. Pan, S.-Y., Litscher, G., (...) Sun J.-N., Ko K.-M. 2014 *Evidence-Based Complementary and Alternative Medicine.* 20 pages	294
'Ethnomedicine'	2,378	The value of plants used in traditional medicine for drug discovery. Fabricant, D.S., Farnsworth, N.R. 2001. *Environmental Health Perspectives* 109 (Suppl 1), pp 69–75	1,407
'Natural medicine'	2,354	Techniques for extraction and isolation of natural products: A comprehensive review. Zhang, Q.-W., Lin, L.-G., Ye, W.-C. 2018 *Chinese Medicine (United Kingdom)* 13(1)	752

(continued)

Table 3.1: Overview of results (continued)

Strings entered	Results	Most cited paper	Citations
'Faith healing'	934	Complementary and alternative medicine use among adults: United States, 2002. Barnes, P.M., Powell-Griner, E., McFann, K., Nahin, R.L. 2004 *Advance Data* (343), pp 1–19	1,442
'Popular medicine'	890	Antioxidant properties of natural compounds used in popular medicine for gastric ulcers. Repetto, M.G., Llesuy, S.F. 2002 *Brazilian Journal of Medical and Biological Research* 35(5), pp 523–34	423
'Indigenous medicine'	531	Sesquiterpene lactones specifically inhibit activation of NF-κB by preventing the degradation of IκB-α and IκB-β. Hehner, S.P., Heinrich, M., Bork, P.M., (...), Dröge, W., Schmitz, M.L. 1998 *Journal of Biological Chemistry* 273(3), pp 1288–97	362
'National medicine'	382	Poor-quality antimalarial drugs in southeast Asia and sub-Saharan Africa. Nayyar, G.M.L., Breman, J.G., Newton, P.N., Herrington, J. 2012 *The Lancet Infectious Diseases* 12(6), pp 488–96	281
'Plant-based medicine'	376	Natural products as α-Amylase and α-Glucosidase inhibitors and their hypoglycaemic potential in the treatment of diabetes: An update. Tundis, R., Loizzo, M.R., Menichini, F. 2010 *Mini-Reviews in Medicinal Chemistry* 10(4), pp 315–31	549
'Religious healing'	205	Varieties of healing. 2: A taxonomy of unconventional healing practices. Kaptchuk, T.J., Eisenberg, D.M. 2001 *Annals of Internal Medicine* 135(3), pp 196–204	125
'Unconventional medicine'	142	Unconventional Medicine in the United States – Prevalence, Costs, and Patterns of Use. Eisenberg, D.M., Kessler, R.C., Foster, C., (...), Calkins, D.R., Delbanco, T.L. 1993 *New England Journal of Medicine* 328(4), pp 246–52	3,664
Nonbiomedical★	77	Hidden reasons some patients visit doctors. Barsky III, A.J. 1981. *Annals of Internal Medicine* 94(4), pp 492–8	181
'Unorthodox medicine'	21	Screening of crude extracts of six medicinal plants used in South-West Nigerian unorthodox medicine for anti-methicillin resistant Staphylococcus aureus activity. Akinyemi, K.O., Oladapo, O., Okwara, C.E., Ibe, C.C., Fasure, K.A. 2005 *BMC Complementary and Alternative Medicine* 5, 6	261

Figure 3.1: Semantic topography of non-biomedical modalities

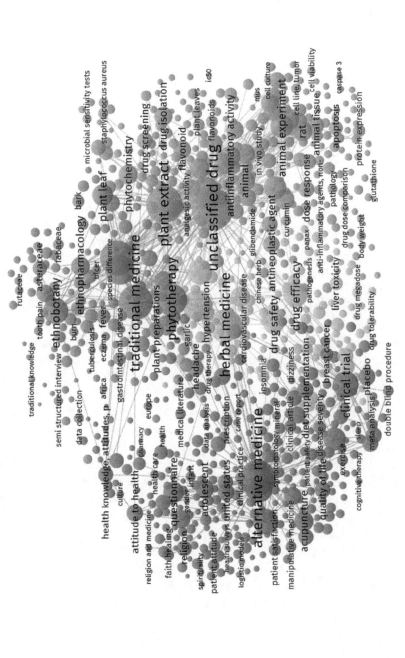

clusters 1–4 are hereafter named after their nodal modalities – their most influential concepts.

The clustering techniques employed were such that cluster membership of each node is probabilistic rather than catergorical (soft clustering), with no subcluster partitioning (flat clustering). Probabilistic clustering represents the assignment of keywords to clusters as probabilities which indicate the likelihood of a data point belonging to a particular cluster, as opposed to 'hard' clustering, where a data point is assigned to a single cluster. This approach enables a more flexible and nuanced representation of keywords' relationships to clusters, especially in scenarios where keywords lie close to the boundary of multiple clusters. We will now do a close reading of each of the knowledge clusters identified through these analytical choices.

Reading of knowledge clusters

Cluster 1: Alternative medicine

Alternative medicine is the most influential concept both within its cluster and within the overall network. It is also the concept with the most associated non-biomedical modalities, namely complementary medicine, complementary therapies, complementary and alternative medicine, integrated medicine, faith healing, holistic care, manipulative medicine, and religious healing. These modalities can be understood as belonging to the same conceptual level; they are umbrella terms that designate therapeutic modalities existing outside of mainstream biomedicine.

This cluster also features terms that describe more specific modalities. These terms include acupuncture, acupressure, allopathy, aromatherapy, Ayurveda, chiropractic, diet therapy, homeopathy, hypnosis, kinesiotherapy, naturopathy, osteopathy, and tai chi. The countries and continents featured in this cluster are Australia, Canada, China, Israel, Japan, the UK, the US, Europe, and Asia. As we shall see later on, this is in stark contrast with the geopolitics associated with unclassified drug and traditional medicine clusters.

Also featured in this cluster are names of disease and condition. These include breast cancer, breast neoplasms, chronic diseases, chronic pain, depression/depressive disorder, fibromyalgia (muscle pain)/low back pain, HIV infections, mental disease & disorders, mood disorder, musculoskeletal disease, and osteoarthritis. It can be seen that some of these diseases and conditions are gendered and aged; some, such as HIV and depression, are more politicized than others.

Alternative medicine research also appears to be very patient-oriented. This is reflected through the presence of keywords such as attitudes, patient satisfaction, surveys, questionnaires, and quality of life in this cluster. This character distinguishes alternative medicine as a conceptual cluster from clusters such as traditional medicine and herbal medicine, which are more disease-oriented and plant-constituent-oriented.

Cluster 2: Unclassified drug

Unclassified drug as a term is in itself a novel finding; it was not included in the original search strings. Unclassified drug encapsulates a distinctly biomedical approach to studying non-biomedical modalities, as it signifies an untamed 'other' that evades the task of scientific ordering. A majority of terms associated with unclassified drug are biochemical, such as acetic acid ethyl ester, antibacterial agent, antidiabetic activity, antifungal agent, artemisinin (antimalarial agent), and hyperglycemia. As such, unclassified drug represents the interests of pharmacology in non-biomedical modalities. This cluster also features the complete scientific process in its set of terms, namely targeting, identifying, evaluating, isolating, screening, and synthesizing drugs for pharmaceutical use. There is no occurrence of terms denoting geographical location anywhere in this cluster; it is as if the workings of biomedical scientific discovery are independent of the geopolitical structure which haunts those who escape laboratories and randomized controlled trials. Two non-biomedical modalities featured in this cluster are natural medicine and Ayurvedic medicine. Natural medicine as a term is emblematic of the nature vs science dichotomy; this is consistent with the overall narrative of the term unclassified drug. The presence of Ayurvedic medicine in this cluster signifies its unique credence in pharmacology. This will be further explored in the Discussion section. The absence of geography descriptors in this cluster suggests that this credence, however, seems to be detached from the larger socio-cultural and political discourse surrounding the legitimacy of medical traditions.

The diseases and conditions associated with unclassified drugs include cancer, diabetes, liver injury, and diseases related to metabolism. Within this cluster, these diseases and conditions are mentioned not only in relation to treatment, but also prevention and protection – particularly with regard to cancer and liver conditions.

Cluster 3: Herbal medicine

Herbal medicine, contrary to unclassified drugs, is firmly grounded in the geopolitics of medical traditions. *Materia medica*, an old-fashioned term that designates the branch of academic study which precedes modern pharmacology (Whyte et al, 2002), is featured in this cluster. Other terms include Ayurvedic drug, Chinese drug/herb/medicine, and traditional Chinese medicine. These terms refer to two medical traditions whose development date back to antiquity and the medieval period, and as such are comparable to European medical systems.

The diseases and traditions associated with herbal medicine include anxiety disorder, cancer (particularly colorectal, lung, and prostate cancer), dementia, fatigue, heart infarction, hypercholesterolemia, hyperlipidemia, insomnia, irritable colon, liver cirrhosis, liver toxicity, malignant neoplastic disease, menopause, obesity, Parkinson's disease, rheumatoid arthritis, sleep disorder, and xerostomia (dry mouth syndrome). There seems to be a more pronounced intersection between age and gender in the diseases within this cluster.

Cluster 4: Traditional medicine

Traditional medicine as a cluster features the highest number of diseases and conditions. These include abdominal pain, allergy, anaemia, arthritis, asthma, backache, bronchitis, influenza/the common cold, constipation, diabetes, diarrhoea, dysentery, dyspepsia (indigestion), eczema (rash), epilepsy, fever, flatulence, gastrointestinal disease, headache, heart disease, haemorrhoid, hepatitis, malaria, migraine, neurologic disease, pneumonia, pruritus (skin itch), respiratory tract disease, tooth pain, and tuberculosis. This is a diverse set of diseases and conditions, which may reflect the semantic malleability of the word 'traditional' within the 'traditional vs modern' dichotomy. This is the only cluster that does not feature cancer in its midst.

Other non-biomedical modalities in this cluster include ethnobotany, ethnomedicine, ethnopharmacology, folk medicine, indigenous knowledge, medicinal plants, traditional knowledge, and African medicine. There is also a diverse set of countries and continents featured in this cluster, including Africa, Brazil, India, Iran, Italy, Mexico, Nigeria, Pakistan, South America, Spain, and Turkey. There is no English-speaking country featured in this collection of geographic descriptors; this is in contrast with those featured in the alternative medicine cluster. Alternative medicine might be a construct more popular to the Anglosphere, where non-biomedical modalities are primarily studied under the framework of integration and/or isolation. By contrast, 'traditional medicine' seems to be used in contexts where integration and isolation are not the sole strategies of meaning-making. In countries where non-biomedical modalities enjoy a less subjugated status, 'traditional' as a substantiator is invoked both as an ode to historical discontinuities and as a political gesture – particularly in the case of postcolonial states and continents, such as India, Pakistan, and Africa.

A way forward: non-biomedical modalities and scholarly knowledge about them

From our close reading of the main semantic map above, we can further identify five main themes of discussion. These themes are: (i) the overall expanding territories of all four knowledge domains; (ii) boundary and proximity of each domain in relation to one another; (iii) the geography of knowledge production in this area; (iv) methodological pitfalls encoded in terms used; and (v) the disconnection of cancer from traditional medicine as a domain. By looking closely at these themes, we can further substantiate our definition of non-biomedical modalities as existing in separation but not isolation from biomedicine – a term much better equipped to reflect the state of literature on medical practices and knowledge at the margin of scientific medical knowledge.

The first theme concerns the **overall upward trend** of all existing terms used to describe non-biomedical modalities in the corpus; despite widespread recognition of the problematic nature of these terms, they continue to be used and referenced across different disciplines. While terms such as alternative medicine, traditional medicine, and herbal medicine have seen their popularity fluctuate over time, they remain the most influential nodes around which knowledge within this domain is organized. This finding resonates with what Daston and Galison (2007) observe to be the surprising longevity of scientific epistemic virtues, in which concepts and methods do not usually replace each other like 'succession of kings' (p 111). They instead accumulate into a repertoire of possible forms of knowing. As long as there are urgent conceptual challenges to the acquisition and securing of knowledge that can be addressed through existing forms of knowing, concepts and methods would not become extinct; they would emerge and evolve. In this sense, knowledge production about non-biomedical modalities within scholarly literature written in the English language resembles problematic networks that span 'webs of interest', which stabilize over time while constantly expanding and adjusting for the sake of their own survival. This process is vital to acquiring knowledge in scientific practices. The biases encoded in these terminologies will most likely carry themselves well into the future; their meanings and connotations, however, will also shift with time as emerging concepts become connected to their networks of meaning.

Foucault (1966) noted in his discussion on naming and representation that when a discourse seizes upon the adjective to designate not only modifications to meanings, but also the very substance of its main propositions, as is the case with the nature of scholarly discourse on non-biomedical modalities, the adjective becomes substantival rather than qualifying. The noun, which would otherwise be articulating substance, behaves like an accident within this discourse; it has become adjectival. Be it traditional, alternative, complementary, herbal, natural, integrative, or indigenous – the adjectives used to describe therapeutic modalities within this knowledge domain seem to overshadow the modalities themselves. One way to disrupt this discourse is to discard the 'adjective + medicine' formula altogether by co-opting the horizontal articulation that has defined the scientific discourse of biomedicine, in favour of the term non-biomedical modalities.

The second theme concerns the **boundaries among different knowledge clusters** within this semantic landscape, as well as their relative proximity to one another. We can see from the map that traditional medicine, herbal medicine, and unclassified drug, together with their associated concepts, are closer to one another than they are to alternative medicine and its associated cluster. This is somewhat counterintuitive, considering how unclassified drug both as a term and as a cluster stands out from the rest of the map semantically: the publications within its population mostly reside within the biomedical domain, feature biochemical jargon, and give no mention of geographical locations. There is a kind of 'placelessness' that sanitizes scientific practices in laboratories. This finding substantiates the original definition of non-biomedical knowledge as existing in separation, but not isolation, from scientific biomedical knowledge. While traditional medicine and herbal medicine attach themselves more closely to unclassified drug, which acts as a bridge between the biomedical domain and its non-biomedical counterpart, alternative medicine seems to have gained a more independent, though not completely secluded, position in relation to the biomedical domain.

From a semantic perspective, this has a number of implications: it is almost as if non-biomedical modalities could claim a more equal footing once they become an 'alternative' to mainstream biomedicine. This signifies a discourse of 'choice' that grants the patient at once the freedom and responsibility to manage their own state of health. This finding also resonates with the ethos of the majority of health-care legislative bodies and subsequent legislations introduced in the West since the late 1970s, including the Dutch Commission on Alternative Systems of Medicine in 1977, the Swedish Minister of Health's Alternative Medicine Committee formed in 1984, the Victorian Parliament Social Development Committee's 'Inquiry into alternative medicine and the health food industry' reporting in 1986 in Australia, the United States Congressional Subcommittee, Subcommittee on Departments of Labor, Health and Human Services, Education, and Related Agencies' hearings on 'Alternative medicine' in 1993; the Norwegian Ministry of Health and Social Affairs' 'Public assessment of alternative medicine' from 1998; House of Lords Select Committee on Science and Technology's report on 'Complementary and alternative medicine' in 2000, the US White House Commission on Complementary and Alternative Medicine's reporting in 2002, and a Ministerial Advisory Committee's report on 'Complementary and alternative health care in New Zealand' for the Minister of Health in 2004. This shift in language use also coincides with what Wahlberg (2007) characterizes as a shift in regulatory discourse in the UK during the closing decades of the 20th century. The battleground of good vs bad medicine has shifted to the ethical domain of practitioner qualification and conduct; it has moved away from the epistemological domain of the late 19th and early 20th centuries as well as the commercial domain of miracle cures and patent medicine of the 18th and 19th centuries (Wahlberg, 2007). This could partially explain the significant wealth of the alternative medicine domain within our map. Alternative medicine is the domain with the most number of publications, the most number of connections, the most bridges that link it to the rest of the map, and is the furthest away from the second wealthiest domain in this landscape – unclassified drug – in an almost polarizing fashion. What Wahlberg (2007) observes to be a turn to the practitioner in the discourse on non-biomedical practices might have evolved to repulse discursive themes that precede this turn. These themes are that of epistemology (with unclassified drugs being a translation operator) and commercial opportunity (with traditional medicine and herbal medicine as translation operators). This also suggests that the ethical and epistemological domains of current scholarly literature on non-biomedical practices seem to have diverged from each other.

The third theme concerns the **geography of knowledge production**, as evidenced in the previous section. Apart from unclassified drug, all other knowledge clusters are firmly grounded in their geographical context. This represents a kind of geographical stickiness which contextualizes knowledge about non-biomedical modalities. While herbal medicine as a cluster is associated exclusively with Ayurvedic and Chinese medicines, alternative medicine is used in literature about the West and Asia. Traditional medicine, on the other hand, is used alongside a more eclectic set of geographical descriptors. Herbal medicine and *materia medica* have a unique evocation of materiality; they encapsulate therapeutic substances that possess exchange value, whose commodity careers are disrupted and displaced by commercially manufactured synthetic drugs. Foundational texts of the Ayurvedic tradition as well as Chinese Shen-nung's scripture on *materia medica* dating from the first millennium of our era both contain hundreds of medicinal recipes and descriptions of therapeutic substances (Unschuld, 1988; Whyte et al, 2002). The spread of biomedical pharmaceuticals to India and China was rapid and far-reaching after World War II; antibiotics were imported to China during the 1950s (Dong et al, 1999), while by the 1960s antibiotics were incorporated in the *materia medica* of Ayurvedic practitioners in India (Taylor, 1976). This materiality also designates the terms and conditions for counterflows; the popularization of Ayurveda in the West has come hand in hand with the reduction of this tradition to a mere supplier of pharmaceutical products – a process Banerjee (2008) describes as the 'pharmaceuticalization' of Ayurveda. In the US, where roughly one in five adults uses herbal medicine, the standardization of complex Chinese herbal formulations has also been substantially linked to the discourse on regulation, efficacy, and safety (Bent, 2008). This narrative mirrors that of 'unclassified drug'.

This narrative of therapeutic materiality does not extend to terms like ethnobotany, ethnomedicine, and ethnopharmacology – which all belong to the traditional medicine cluster. This is our fourth theme of discussion – that of a **methodological nature**. Whyte et al (2002) observe that ethnopharmacology as a field focuses on the biochemical properties and effects of indigenous medicines while accounting for people's own conception about these modalities, whereas ethnomedicine as an approach places primary value on contextualization. Studies conducted using this approach usually situate therapeutic modalities within the cosmology, ritual, and knowledge of particular ethnic groups. Whyte et al (2002) argue that a major weakness of ethnomedicine is its presentation of context as integrated tradition; this is an analytical move that portrays culture and society as static and homogenous. It is no coincidence, then, that these terms are clustered around 'traditional medicine'. 'Traditional medicine' carries a sense of fixity that stabilizes pre-modern cultures of therapy as rigid and unchanging, while simultaneously being disorderly and excessively repetitive. This conceptualization opens up the possibilities of scientific innovation and disruption. Confined to a discourse constructed on an opaque temporality, traditional medicine and its associated *ethno-x* are caught in an intricate web of contextual sense-making that seems to absolve them of their materiality.

This brings us to our last theme of discussion, which concerns the **disconnection of cancer from the traditional medicine cluster**. As mentioned in the previous section, traditional medicine is the only cluster in which no occurrence of 'cancer' or any variation thereof is included in the current map. This does not mean that there exists no publication in the dataset wherein 'cancer' and 'traditional medicine' occur together; these terms do not, however, co-occur with a frequency significant enough for their relationship to be represented on the map.

Cancer is a disease as old as tradition itself; ancient Greek medical treatises of tumour formation and its therapeutic methods date back to the Hippocratic corpus and Galenic medicine (Karpozilos and Pavlidis, 2004). The word 'tumour' (瘤) in Chinese appeared in prehistoric cave carvings in North-West China as far back as 1000BC, while a more technical word for tumour (癌) appeared around 1200AD, describing ulcerative lumps and occurrences of sinuses and fistulae (Li, 1996; Bao et al, 2006; Leung et al, 2007). Ayurvedic classics developed an elaborate vocabulary to describe cancer, with *granthi* referring to minor neoplasm and *arbuda* referring to major neoplasm. They also used a range of terms to refer to benign neoplasm (*vataja*, *pittaja*, and *kaphaja*) and malignant tumours (*tridosaja*) (Balachandran and Govindarajan, 2005). Despite its old age, cancer is an increasingly technologized disease. Since the 1970s, biomedical diagnosis of cancer has been infused with modern technologies, thanks to significant progress made in ultrasound (sonography), computed tomography (CT scans), magnetic resonance imaging (MRI scans), and positron emission tomography (PET scans). As a result, biomedical treatment of cancer has grown to include technologically sophisticated methods such as cryosurgery (the use of liquid nitrogen spray to freeze and kill cancer cells), the use of lasers to cut the tumour tissue of cervix, larynx, liver, rectum, skin, and other organs, chemotherapy, hormonal therapy, radiation therapy, and immunotherapy (Sudhakar, 2009). Progress in cancer nanotechnology promises advances in early detection, diagnostics, and prognostics, as well as more targeted treatment with nanovectors and more precision in the patterning of surfaces with imaging moieties (Halappanavar et al, 2018). Biomedical technologies, through magnifying the 'visibility' of cancer, exercise a kind of panoptic disciplinary power that fixes a space for the disease as dwelling inside the body. This is a space juxtaposed to other spaces – a body-technological space.

Tradition, deriving from the Latin word *tradere*, meaning 'to hand over' or 'deliver', originally referred to the passing on of knowledge or doctrine. The word therefore had an original emphasis on the process of distribution; this meaning, however, was slipped into a more static focus on what was being distributed as tradition became associated with issues of right, duty, authority, and respect (Scheid, 2007). Traditions have the ability to assert historical continuity as a sense of connection with the past through repetition of norms, values, and behaviours. The invention of tradition, however, is an activity that persists well into modernity. The products of this invention are 'responses to novel situations which take the form of reference to old situations, or which establish their own past by quasi-obligatory repetition' (Hobsbawm and Ranger, 2012, p 2). The decoupling of cancer and traditional medicine might owe itself to the highly technologized conditions under which the disease itself becomes understood in scholarly literature.

Notes on limitations of analysis

There are three main limitations with the semantic mapping of literature conducted in this chapter. Firstly, the mapping was conducted on a corpus of the most cited scientific publications in the field of TM/CAM indexed by Scopus, generated through the use of 18 search terms collected from a qualitative review of literature. The corpus is an artefact constructed from these systematic analytical choices, and as such operationalizes a discourse found in the specific literature retrieved. Although containing a substantial number of records (over 33,000 articles), the corpus is not exhaustive. Secondly, the current corpus only includes English-language scholarly articles. English-language literature is by far the most systematically recorded body of literature through large databases, which enable the structured querying, retrieval, and processing necessary for co-word analysis. However, there is space for future research to incorporate non-English literature into a similar semantic analysis. Finally, there might be merit in conducting systematic mapping of literature using multiple databases for comparative and complementary purposes. In addition to Scopus, future research might incorporate literature retrieved from other indexing services, such as Web of Science and Google Scholar. Even though Google Scholar is the only 'big data' academic literature system to date with highly extensive coverage, it is also the most limited in its capacity to export bibliometric data, and also the most opaque in indexing mechanism. Google Scholar's strict query rate limits, proprietary ranking algorithm, and lack of a master list of sources are major barriers to sustainable data mining using this service.

Miracle cures as non-biomedical modalities

By employing a network approach, this chapter has mapped the various terms in the literature on non-biomedical modalities into four clusters: alternative medicine, unclassified drugs, herbal medicine, and traditional medicine. The map produced here is original in that it is data-driven; it is different from existing, qualitatively constructed classifications and taxonomies in that it relies very little on interpretation. As such, the current approach does not leave a lot of room for nuance. Instead, it is a precursor to interpretation; counting and probabilistic modelling are useful insofar as a large amount of data is handled efficiently, whose themes can be shown with high reliability and replicability. The clustering presented in this chapter claims to neither be definitive nor exhaustive. It is, however, a rigorous map with which to navigate the highly complex and interdisciplinary literatures on non-biomedical traditions and practices.

It should be abundantly clear by now that terminologies are not value-free conventions of speech. Terminological utterance spins webs of meanings that presuppose the act of saying itself, whose convergence and intersection reflect and reshape academic discourse as it produces its subject. This chapter suggests that non-biomedical modalities, defined as therapeutic modalities that exist in separation but not isolation from biomedicine, is a term much better equipped to reflect the current state of literature on therapeutic modalities that exist at the margin of scientific medicine. While the term itself does not resolve issues of power imbalance that exist between the scientific and the non-scientific, it helps bring these issues to the fore. The term also better captures the historical disruption that biomedicine both as a scientific discipline and as a mechanism of body surveillance came to solidify modernity around the world. The term therefore highlights the interaction between 'bio' and 'medicine' through the invisible hyphen that no longer seems to separate the two; it serves to remind us that biomedicine and its technologies are a very specific, and rather recent, episode in the history of medicine. Through its visible hyphen, however, the term highlights the continuity of medical practices that persist at the margin of the scientific enterprise as they continue to evolve and transform themselves through their interaction with biomedicine. It is through this duality that the term non-biomedical invites a critical mode of engagement that might otherwise be easily overlooked – one that allows science to further its commitment to fidelity to the nature of its subject.

This chapter has made the case for understanding miracle cures as non-biomedical modalities. Despite their many mutations across time and context, both in response to the biomedical and in reference to other non-biomedical modalities, miracle cures have continued to proliferate and sustain scholarly interest. This tenet is crucial for the project at hand, which seeks to trace the continuity of medical practices that persist at the margin of the scientific enterprise in the presence of digital technologies – both in praxis and in scholarly knowledge production about praxis. Viewed through this lens, written miracle cure recipes and livestreamed videos of miracle healing are not so much symptoms of a new information disorder as they are digital expressions of historical practices. As these historical practices interact with digital technologies, they not only transform themselves to adapt with the digital milieu, but also significantly transform the temporal and spatial structures of the everyday. In Part II, we will interrogate the digitality of the written form, what this means for the proliferation of written miracle recipes on Facebook, and explore how the logic of digitality can be mobilized towards large-scale analysis of miracle recipes.

Written Networks of Digital Miracles

Prologue: Writings on a wall

Can digital miracles be formalized? What sort of effects does formalization have on the performance of digital miracles? The migration of our dominant written culture onto social media is enabling the digital codification of existing bodies of miraculous cures, allowing them to take on network-like expressions. This digital codification through the written word is an instance of the formalization of digital record-keeping and record-making within the structuring and formatting of social media data architecture. The digitality of writing lends itself to a swathe of computational manipulation, which has been developed both in response to and as a historical result of late 20th-century computationalism. By examining this digitality firstly through a historical lens and subsequently using the tools that have been developed as part of our computational *zeitgeist*, we can begin to examine how written networks of miracle cures on social media might differ from – or resemble – pre-digital organizations and enactments of miracles.

4

Crowd Digitization of Miracle Cures and the Digitality of Writing

That miracle cures became inscribed – that is, committed to space – turned out to be a transformative development. When *Tuệ Tĩnh* composed *Nam Dược Thần Hiệu* [Miraculous Drugs of the South] in Chinese script while living in exile in China, he ended up producing a text that is a blend of a herbal handbook and a pragmatic guide (see Chapter 2). Commonly understood as *Tuệ Tĩnh*'s effort to elucidate Vietnamese medicine to his host country, *Nam Dược Thần Hiệu* was the first text to systematize the use of Vietnamese medicaments within the parameters of Chinese drug theory, so that 'Southern' medicine could be presented to physicians at the Ming court. By way of inscription, miracle cures became subject to decontextualization. By isolating miracle cures from the broader context in which they originally appeared and attempting to abstract away principles about the miracles of the South towards a more generalized and theoretical understanding, *Tuệ Tĩnh* had mobilized an analytical mindset made possible by a culture of literacy which, in 14th-century Vietnam, was populated by the educated elite. The written form is abstracted from matter and in need of explication; they are residues of what has been called 'context-free' language (Hirsch, 1977, p 21) or 'autonomous' discourse (Olson, 1980, p 187). Writing has since the beginning enhanced the primary orality of language, enabling not only the organization of principles of oratory, but also giving rise to the written composition, which further cemented the importance of the analytical mindset – which is intent on pulling things apart, breaking down the dense continuum of experience, and processing information in meaningful segments (Ong, 2002).

Inscription also makes miracle cures portable, even if not contextually transferrable. Copies of '*Nam Dược Thần Hiệu*' were sent back to Vietnam via a diplomatic mission and were kept in the Vietnamese royal libraries prior to the Ming invasion in 1407, even as they were produced for the benefit of the Ming court (see Chapter 2). The fixation of miracle cures on paper was made in assistance of military conquest and colonization; even when *Tuệ Tĩnh* foregrounded a physical and spiritual relationship between Vietnamese people and the land where they live ('Vietnamese medicine for Vietnamese people'), the inscription of miracle cures was meant to assist the Ming with overcoming the 'miasmic climate' of Vietnam as a 'deadly barrier' that set limits for military garrisons and Han settlements. Writing gives thoughts different contours from orally sustained thoughts; crucial to orality, memorable thoughts were thinkable not so much as 'facts', but rather as reflections, often inviting further reflections by the paradoxes they involved (Ong, 2002). The written thought is constrained not only by the written form, but also by formats. Format specifications govern the transference of data structures from one medium to another at the point of contact between human, symbol, and machine (Tenen, 2017). Words that appear on the screen might be functionally similar to those on paper, but they are substantially different. Tenen (2017) argues that computational media complicate our ability to situate inscription; screens as sites of projection that emanate from hidden storage media reveal digital texts that have passed through multiple filters and transformations, such that digital inscription is stratified across multiple incongruent planes. When miracle cures become digitally inscribed, they lend themselves to a range of computational analysis developed both in service of, and in response to, the digital textual environment.

This chapter discusses the crowd digitization of traditional healing recipes from different Vietnamese traditions, namely Northern medicine (*thuốc Bắc*), Southern medicine (*thuốc Nam*), and family recipes (*thuốc gia truyền*). Once kept within families of traditional medical doctors through oral traditions or written up on paper and sold for a fee, these recipes are now shared, discussed, and debated across social media networks on a much larger scale. Social media 'content' – a term reminiscent of the mass media era – comes in a variety of forms, such as machine-readable texts, photos, and videos. These units of content are constrained by platform affordances so that they can be automatically mined and retrieved for analysis *post hoc*. Of these formats, machine-readable text is by far the most computation-friendly, lending itself to automated data manipulation, measuring, and analysis. This is both a symptom of our writing society – that which is saturated with traces of written objects – and a reflection of the digitality of writing. The chapter contextualizes the crowd digitization of miracle cures on Vietnamese Facebook within a longer history of inscription by firstly discussing the emergence of the writing society alongside the digitality of writing, focusing on the implications they have on the mobility and systematization of miracle cures. The chapter continues with a discussion on the rise of the computational text through and with programmable media, as well as the conditions of possibility for computational methods at the intersection of hardware and software. The chapter ends with a mini media archaeology of the written miracle cure, from *Tuệ Tĩnh*'s early attempt to codify Vietnamese 'miraculous cures' in *Hán* script (using Chinese characters) to the contemporary Facebook post format in *chữ quốc ngữ* (Vietnamese Romanized script).

The rise of the writing society and the digitality of writing

How did we come to value abstract and analytical thinking over situational and participatory modes of thought? Walter J. Ong (2002) traces this shift to the rise of literacy and the impact it has on our collective cognitive functions by contrasting cultures of orality and cultures of literacy. The lack of textual permanence and a reliance on memory in societies built around orality mean that people are primed to think memorable thoughts made to be passed on through oral tradition and communal sharing of knowledge, keeping knowledge embedded in the human lifeworld and within a context of struggle. Literacy, on the other hand, allows for the preservation and transmission of knowledge across time and space through the written text; this encourages individuals to form detachment from their immediate experience and separates the knower from the known. When *Tuệ Tĩnh* was made to codify his knowledge of *thuốc Nam* (Southern medicine) in Chinese script and within the parameters laid out by the Ming court, the exercise was extractivistic in nature: the turning of situated knowledge into scripted information marks the start of the political economy of the written text, one that was to be thoroughly technologized with the advent of print and computation centuries later.

This is not to say that the literate thought has completely replaced oral modes of thought, however. Orality serves important communication functions in society, and thus continues to coexist with the written form even in highly literate societies. Residual orality, argues Ong (2002), has a range of different manifestations. In chirographic cultures – cultures that place high value on penmanship and handwriting – residual orality could be assessed in terms of the amount of memorization the culture's educational procedures require (Ong, 2002). Writing about a 'literate orality' that exists within the secondary oral culture induced by radio and television, Ong (2002, pp 156–7) urges future researchers to look into the psychodynamics of orality in relation to the psychodynamics of writing in contexts where people are rapidly moving from total orality to literacy, as well as residually oral subcultures in dominantly high-literacy societies. Readers whose norms and expectancies for formal discourse are governed by a residually oral mindset, for example, relate to a text quite differently from readers whose sense of style is radically textual. That *Tuệ Tĩnh* did not adhere to Chinese classifications based on the Chinese Five Phases (which explains changes in the cosmos in the overcoming and succession of earth, wood, metal, fire, and water in an immutable cycle) was significant. *Tuệ Tĩnh* grouped his pharmaceuticals together according to naturally occurring, easily observable physical similarities – something that could not only be read as an indication of a certain Vietnamese independence of thought regarding the natural world (per Thompson, 2017a), but also as a manifestation of residual orality within *Nam Dược Thần Hiệu* [Miraculous Drugs of the South].

Using the example of the Latin language, which he characterizes as being 'chirographically controlled', Ong (2002, pp 159–60) argues that a literary text in Latin, however complex, and however learnedly understood, was bound to be opaque by comparison with a text in one's own mother's tongue. A mother's tongue, argues Ong (2002, p 160), is always 'written out of a richer mix of unconscious and conscious elements'. Also making a distinction between human languages and computer languages along these lines, Ong (2002, p 7) argues that computer languages are 'forever totally unlike human languages' in that they do not grow out of the unconscious, but directly out of consciousness, where the rules and grammar are stated first and thereafter used – whereas the grammar in natural human languages are abstracted from usage and stated explicitly in words only with difficulty, and never completely.

Inscribing miracle cures: ideographic beginnings

What kind of change did writing bring about for the miracle cures of Vietnam? The inscription of Vietnamese miracle cures was deeply entangled in the geopolitics of the technologies of writing, which in the case of Vietnam involved the colonial powers of China and France. Chinese characters were used to record elements of the Vietnamese language as early as the 8th century (DeFrancis, 1977; Thompson, 1988), and the earliest extant Chinese texts written by Vietnamese dated around the end of the 10th century (Hannas, 1997). Using Chinese characters to record non-Chinese languages was not peculiar to Vietnam; the same process also happened in Japan and Korea. This process was done across Vietnamese, Japanese, and Korean languages through three main strategies: (i) using Chinese characters to semantically represent indigenous words with the same or nearly the same meaning, in which case one would look at a character and read off a native sound corresponding to the word in one's own language; (ii) using Chinese characters for their phonetic value, where one would pick a character that sounded in Chinese like the pronunciation of the target word, and read it as such with the meaning of the indigenous homonym as the one intended; and (iii) Chinese characters were used to represent Sinitic vocabulary borrowed into the indigenous language, in which case the assignment was both semantic and phonetic (Hannas, 1997). The application of Chinese characters in Vietnam resulted in two systems of writing: *chữ Nôm* ('Southern writing') – an ideographic Vietnamese vernacular script generally considered to be uncouth, and *chữ Nho* ('writing of the scholars') – which was the classical Chinese used in literature, correspondence among the literati, and official documents (Hannas, 1997).

DeFrancis (1977) used the term Sino-Vietnamese (*Hán-Việt*) to describe anything written in classical Chinese by a Vietnamese and pronounced, when read aloud, in the Vietnamese manner. What's interesting about Sino-Vietnamese literature is that, on paper, a piece of Sino-Vietnamese literature would be indistinguishable from a piece of Chinese literature; however, when read aloud, a Vietnamese reader would pronounce the Chinese characters with the phonology of their own language (DeFrancis, 1977). The separation of the intellectual elite and the illiterate masses in Vietnam was, however, enforced by Sino-Vietnamese. Ordinary Vietnamese people were not only unable to read anything written in Sino-Vietnamese, but were also unable to understand it even if it was read aloud to them (DeFrancis, 1977).

Despite this 'Chinese wall of foreign writing' (DeFrancis, 1977, p 20), Vietnamese people were united by a common spoken language, with which a body of oral literature consisting of legends, stories, satires, maxims, and folk songs of great antiquity were created and passed along from generation to generation. Unlike the generally stuffy writings of Confucian scholars in Sino-Vietnamese, oral literature was lively, earthy, and biting. This cultural legacy gave rise to the development of *chữ Nôm* – a complex form of demotic writing developed out of the base Chinese script. *Chữ Nôm* has the appearance of Chinese yet is not Chinese, consisting of two main categories of characters. The first category is made up of simple borrowings from Chinese for their phonetic value to represent Vietnamese words with similar or the same sound, and the second category comprises a significant number of 'composite creations' (DeFrancis, 1977, p 25), where new *Nôm* characters were made by combining two Chinese characters. As a result, *chữ Nôm* was neither consistently semantic nor consistently phonetic; the significance of *chữ Nôm*, however, was that 'even illiterates could understand the *Nôm* literature [which] influenced the way it was written. Books had to be composed not to be read but to be recited. And in order for the contents to be remembered after learning, versified form, with its rhythm and its rhyme, virtually imposed itself' (DeFrancis, 1977, p 46). The indigenousness of *chữ Nôm* marginalized its applicability in the eyes of the literati, whose group identity rested in large part in their knowledge of classical Chinese – which commands their position within the Vietnamese social hierarchy (Hannas, 1997).

Chữ Nôm is the script with which *thuốc gia truyền* (family recipes) – a body of knowledge that was passed on within 'medical families' who earned the majority of their livelihood from practising medicine or pharmacy – was composed (Thompson, 2017b). *Thuốc gia truyền* often exhibit ancient Vietnamese ideas about human health and the natural world, and many of them contain at least some admixture of theories from China (Thompson, 2017b). Many of these family recipes before the 1920s have no specified author – a fact Thompson (2017b) attributed to the repression of *chữ Nôm* by the *Nguyễn* dynasty – such that the authors' identities can be protected while circumscribing the communities that can produce such texts as familial. Handwritten in *chữ Nôm* and presenting prescriptions for commonly encountered ailments, *thuốc gia truyền* are primarily concerned with instructions on how to find, recognize, and prepare *materia medica* as practical advice for treatment of everyday illnesses. Despite periods of revival under the 18th-century *Tây Sơn* dynasty with significant headway in poetry – as well as a period of renaissance within the *thuốc gia truyền* genre from the 1920s to at least the 1990s (Thompson, 2017b) – *chữ Nôm* was eventually displaced by *chữ quốc ngữ* – the Romanized Vietnamese script.

Romanization as tokenization: the digitality of writing

Missionary activity by French, Italian, Spanish, and Portuguese priests in Vietnam dated back to the early 17th century, and missionaries were deeply involved in the acquisition of spoken Vietnamese in service of sermon delivery. The study of Vietnamese became an important part of the training for missionary work in Vietnam, and literary tools such as orthographies based on Latin letters and dictionaries soon became an indispensable facilitator of this training (DeFrancis, 1977). Drawing on works by Portuguese missionaries Gaspar d'Amaral and Antonio Barbosa, French Jesuit missionary Alexandre de Rhodes published the first trilingual Vietnamese–Portuguese–Latin dictionary in 1651 in Rome. Even though the Romanized writing system was fairly well-known in the Catholic community, there was little evidence of wide usage until French annexation of Vietnam in 1861.

The transition to alphabetic writing in Vietnam happened comparatively early – that is, before literacy was widespread and before the language had acquired modern Sinitic terms that contributed to ambiguity in the other East Asian languages, such as Japanese and Korean (Hannas, 1997). *Chữ quốc ngữ* is analytical in the sense that it has close ties to the spoken language and is able to capture dialectal differences without sacrificing motivation or accuracy, while lending itself to conventional word processing equipment and programs that were being built for alphabetic characters. That the Vietnamese language itself was, and to some extent continues to be, supported by two other well-developed languages – French and English – created favourable conditions for *chữ quốc ngữ* to have enough breathing space to establish itself gradually and on its own terms (Hannas, 1997).

Hannas (1997) remarks that to the untrained eye, *chữ quốc ngữ* might appear 'cluttered' due to the use of diacritics for special letters and another set of diacritics to indicate tone – resulting in a script that is largely phonemic, posing challenges for typing on 'standard' keyboards. While *chữ quốc ngữ* might have made the Vietnamese language more amenable to computerization, its syllable-based orthography means that words are poorly distinguished in Vietnamese because the preceding ideographic writing systems did not require it. While the concept of a 'word' is notoriously problematic in linguistics in general, the lack of well-defined word division in the Vietnamese language means that intimate knowledge of word-building habits and basic meaningful forms is often required for the task of word identification. In Vietnamese, the syntactic units which are capable of being uttered independently or combined freely are not always monosyllables, but often sequences of two or more syllables. For example, while some monosyllabic words have meanings in themselves (for example, *thích* means to like), a large number of words are made up of monosyllabic types (for example, *giải thích* means to explain; *thích nghi* means to adapt). About 85 per cent of Vietnamese word types are composed of at least two syllables, and more than 80 per cent of syllable types are words by themselves (Le et al, 2008; Thang et al, 2008).

These seemingly obscure linguistic details have profound implications for computation. In automated natural language processing (NLP), for example, the automated breaking down of sentences into individual words – also known as tokenization – could be accomplished quite straightforwardly by splitting apart words whenever there is a space between them. While tokenizing by space works well for English, it does not work for languages like Vietnamese. Computation works off the logic of distinction, decision, difference, and division (Galloway, 2014); at the heart of the digitality of computation is an underlying homogeneity produced out of standardization, prefabrication, and repetition. This is in contrast with the analogue paradigm, which requires an underlying heterogeneity where 'the stuff of the world remains unaligned, idiosyncratic, singular' (Galloway, 2014, p 103). It is in this sense that digitality is more than just the binary of zeros and ones; digitality is about turning one into two – about the making distinct of atoms and making uniform of dissimilar ingredients. Digitization, as such, is a process whereby unorganized and uncoded aggregates of things become fixed and aligned through routines, procedures, regularities, and spatial architectures (Galloway, 2014). The condition of the digital is that of separation, alienation, distinction, division, and making discrete (Galloway, 2014).

The digital text is always already simulated, for it emerges out of a radical standardization at the atomic level. Semantic aspects of communication were famously considered irrelevant to the engineering of communication, per Claude Shannon,[1] because communication systems were to be designed so that they could operate across all possible communication instances. From a computational point of view, the written text becomes a selection from a field of definable alternatives – and literary corpuses sources of data to be read not closely but probabilistically (Franklin, 2015). Insofar as programming is also a form of alphabetization, the arithmetic exposes language as a form of medium (Griffin et al, 1996). What can be captured through literary means, as such, is also amenable to the imposition of a digital worldview. To the extent that the medium of writing not only carries 'content' – and content of one medium is always another medium (Kittler, 1996) – but also couples storage and transmission, digital inscription gives rise to all sociotechnical artifacts that computers mediate. While the printed word is governed by laws from without, the digital text is governed by code from within; in very important ways, the digital text is always already code in the sense that it is always parsed and potentially executable (Tenen, 2017). For Galloway (2014, p 55), at the core of Western thought is a digitality that makes it possible to think about the instance alongside the transcendental, form alongside matter, media alongside comprehension, life alongside authenticity, writing alongside originality – and never one without the other.

The crowd digitization of miracle cures, as we will see later in this chapter, does much more than simply turning the handwritten and printed text into digitally encoded text that appears on the screen. As the written text becomes digitized, language becomes programmable; as language itself becomes automated, it becomes even further removed from its context. The feeling of material transcendence in the digital text, argues Tenen (2017), is tied directly to the underlying physical affordances of electromagnetic storage – which gives the digital text an ephemeral quality that does not exist in the physicality of ink on paper or inscriptions on stone. Physicality grounds words in a specific time and place, whereas the digital text can appear and disappear in an instant, rendering it both omnipresent and evanescent. Text as code renders not only the alphabetic text, but also images, algorithmic. As we will see in Part III, the algorithmic rendering of time and space also has significant implications for miracle cure practices.

From paper to electromagnetic storage: the materiality of writing

The conversion of natural languages into electric signals saw the languages of people and machines enter the same mixed communications stream, paving the way for the automation of language (Tenen, 2017). The reduction of diverse human language scripts to a set of discrete, regularized, and reliably reproducible characters allows communication messages to be sent over great distances and makes it possible to program machines remotely; as soon as human languages were translated into machine-transmittable code, automated technologies and systems were put in place so that machines could communicate with other machines without human intervention. Human-compatible alphabets and machine control code became intimately coupled; the stabilization of programming languages to control machines means that content for people is now routinely intermixed with code (Tenen, 2017). Such is the condition for the rise of programmable media: writing becomes less about making marks on paper, and more about simulation on the computer screen. Texts that appear on the screen are redoubled and ephemeral; their enduring form resides as traces in computer memory that are legible only to those with the specialized tools and training necessary to decipher them (Tenen, 2017). It is in this sense that the logic of automated analysis rests on the level of programmable media, whose epistemology is rooted in cellular arrays of discrete entities divided and subdivided into systems and subsystems.

The digital text passes through layers of transformation before it could emerge at the surface: the inscriptions we see on the liquid crystal screen are visual projections that emanate from hidden storage media of magnetic pulse and circuit state, rendering the digital inscription contingent and malleable. The current textual condition that we find ourselves in, argues Tenen (2017), rests on the three-fold essential architecture that took shape in the late 1960s: programmable media, electromagnetic storage, and screen. The digital text is sealed hermetically and hermeneutically (that is, in ways that are recalcitrant to human interpretation) inside solid-state storage before it appears in a human-compatible fashion on screen. The computer memory, where computing instructions are executed by a control unit via a program counter that keeps track of the memory address of the next instruction for execution, is part of what has come to be known as the von Neumann[2] architecture deployed in most modern computers. In von Neumann terms, an input-output unit allows the computer to interact with the outside world, and both data and instructions are stored in the same memory address space – so that program instructions and data can be fetched from and written to memory using the same set of instructions (the 'stored-program'). It is in the temporary home of the computer memory that words can be manipulated – modified, erased, rewritten – at the point of (re)inscription. For Tenen (2017), this represents a step change in the conditions of the written text: it has entered a complex system of executable code and inscrutable control instruction, wherein its material lightness came at the price of legibility. The screen as a site of simulation might emulate the many familiar analogue forms of engagement with the written word, such as bookmarking, highlighting, page turning, marginalia, and so on – all while concealing the material properties that give the illusion of static text despite the dynamic properties of projection, which have brought texts closer to the moving image.

This newly gained proximity to the moving image poses important questions about media form and format in relation to text. The modality of information – text, sound, or image – has profound implications on the substantive content being communicated, and their convergence on the digital device as well as automated communication systems has transformed our collective information environment. The text now routinely appears alongside sound and the moving image in composite arrangements that are mediated through data structures that operate according to predefined rules; it is in this sense that data formats transform both an object's physical properties and its ideational subject matter (Tenen, 2017). The alphanumeric universality of computers enables an environment for the propagation of sociocollective knowledge about numerous topics often in forms that contravene the conventions and narrative structures of books. The digitization of non-biomedical knowledge by means of social media discussion groups, for example, does not simply replicate what has been said, inscribed in handwritten notes, or printed in bounded books. Digitization has made possible new expressions of information and knowledge, often as amalgamations of previous media forms – as the next section will demonstrate.

Crowd digitization of miracle cures: a mini media archaeology of written miracles

That *Nam Dược Thần Hiệu* [Miraculous Drugs of the South] was not printed in Vietnam until 1761 despite the existence of its copies in Vietnam prior to the Ming invasion in 1407 is often attributed to the success of another work by *Tuệ Tĩnh*, written prior to his exile in China and in the demotic *Nôm* script, *Hồng Nghĩa Giác Tư Y Thư* [Medical Books by Hong Nghia] (Monnais et al, 2011). This work had become a standard practical medical reference for Vietnamese traditional healers long before it was presented to the royal court of the *Lê* dynasty (1428–1788) in 1717 (Monnais et al, 2011). *Nam Dược Thần Hiệu* [Miraculous Drugs of the South] was not printed in Vietnam until 1761. Surviving copies of these woodblock prints are kept in the National Library of Vietnam and digitized copies are hosted by the Nôm Preservation Foundation (see Figure 4.1). The text was translated into Vietnamese and printed in *chữ quốc ngữ* (Romanized script) for the first time in 1960 by the now defunct *Viện Nghiên cứu Đông y* [Eastern Medicine Research Institute] (That Son, 2016); the second edition of *Nam Dược Thần Hiệu* [Miraculous Drugs of the South] in *chữ quốc ngữ* was published in 1972 as a series of 11 books (Suc Khoe Doi Song, 2022).

The significance of Buddhist temples as key sites of print culture in Vietnam prior to French colonization is well documented (Baldanza, 2018; Nguyen et al, 2018). That *Tuệ Tĩnh* was a Buddhist monk whose milieu was grounded in a constellation of communities, institutions, texts, and

Figure 4.1: Sample pages of *Nam Dược Thần Hiệu* in *Hán* script (woodblock print), digitized by Nôm Preservation Foundation

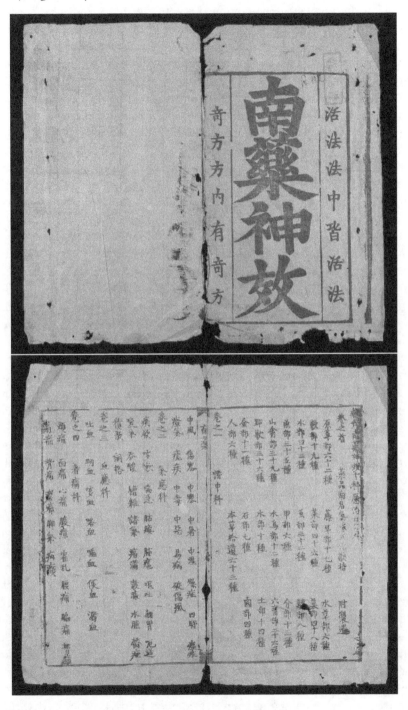

practices strongly influenced by the Buddhist tradition not only had an impact on his approach to pharmacopeia, but arguably also on the forms in which the knowledge he compiled became fossilized and subsequently disseminated. The handwritten word has an intimate relationship with the printed word not only in the sense that the movable type mechanized what could have been achieved by hand on paper, but also in that their forms are often interchangeable. Studying some 80 texts collected from *Thắng Nghiêm* and *Phổ Nhân* temples in Northern Vietnam, Baldanza (2018) found that *Hán-Nôm* literary culture continued, especially within Buddhist and medical circles, well into the 1940s – and that where printed versions of popular texts fell short to meet demand, handwritten copies often acted as substitutes especially for people who could not find or afford a personal copy. In this lively book economy, popular texts such as *Nam Dược Thần Hiệu* [Miraculous Drugs of the South] would be edited, abridged, annotated, and reprinted many times, putting several different versions into simultaneous circulation.

From the *Phổ Nhân* temple collection, several copies of *Nam Dược Thần Hiệu* [Miraculous Drugs of the South] survived both in print and in handwritten manuscript; a curious version of this text which was included in the collection is the *Tân San Nam Dược Thần Hiệu Thập Khoa Ứng Trị* 新刊南藥神效十科應治 [Newly Cut Miraculous Medicines of the South, Remedies from the Ten Branches] – a reprint of the original *Nam Dược Thần Hiệu* [Miraculous Drugs of the South]. The phrase 'newly cut' (*tân san* 新刊) is a clear reference to the medium of the woodblock print, and yet there are several handwritten copies of this version in the collection (see Figure 4.2). From the handwritten *gia truyền* [family recipes] – which are kept within generations of medical families or sold for a fee – to handwritten copies of bibliographic volumes, there is a stickiness in how the pre-digitized word moves as inscription precisely because of the flat distinction between form and content, wherein the space between type and page is practically non-existent. On the other hand, the flatness of digital inscription is but an illusion: ideas about form, content, style, letter, and word transform as texts move from paper to pixel (Drucker, 2001; Hayles, 2004; McGann, 2016). The perpetual transfiguration between screen and electromagnetic storage that happens in the background in order for the digital text to function has transformed our contemporary textual condition – and enabled the proliferation of digital discourse networks not only as content, but also as emerging forms of sociality.

If the modern printing press made it possible for books to routinely include illustrations – hand-drawn or digitally designed (see Figure 4.3) – alongside the static text, then the affordances of social media made it possible for the digital text to reveal its dynamic qualities. Facebook users routinely share photos alongside text caption not only so that their posts have a better chance of showing up on their network contacts' feeds (Facebook's dynamic

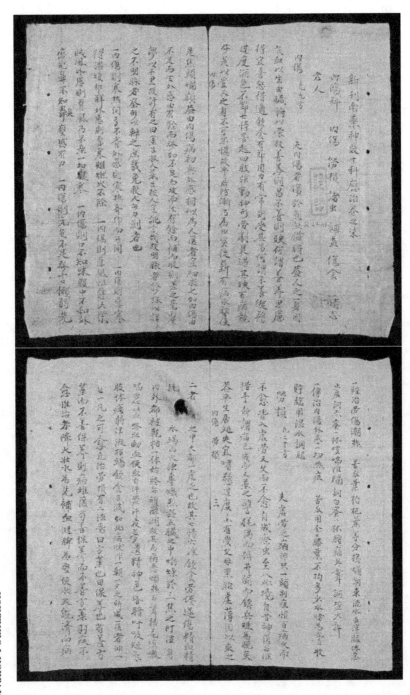

Figure 4.2: Sample pages of *Tân San Nam Dược Thần Hiệu Thập Khoa Ứng Trị* (handwritten copies of woodblock print), digitized by Nôm Preservation Foundation

Figure 4.3: Sample pages of *Nam Dược Thần Hiệu In Chữ Quốc Ngữ* (Romanized script), digitized and made publicly available by Ninh Thuận province public library

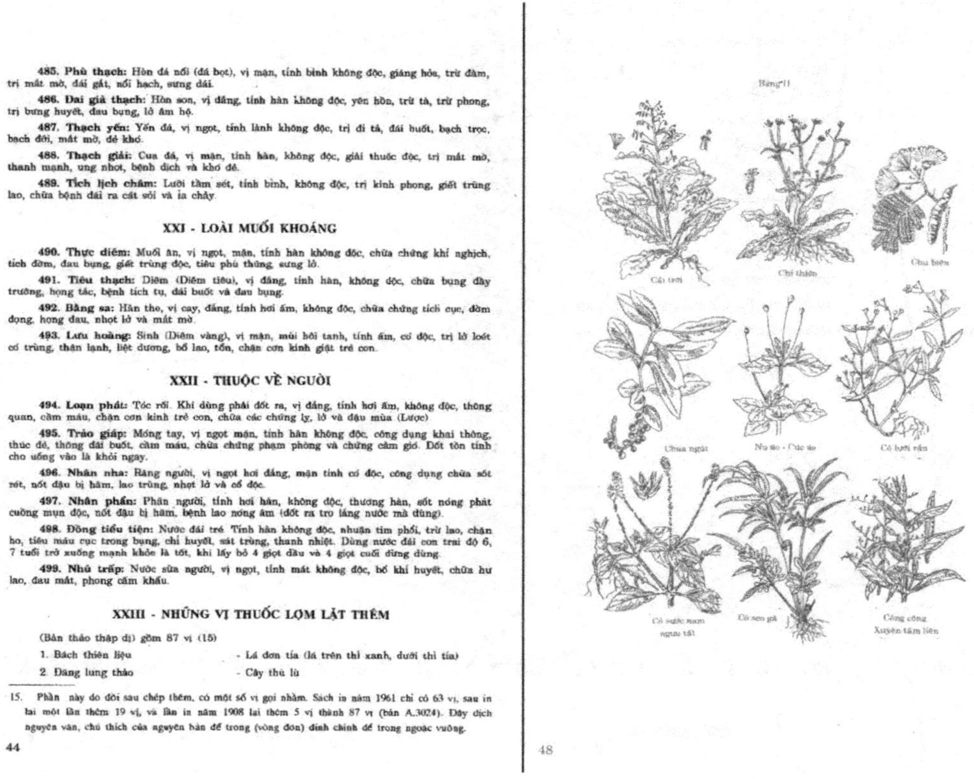

485. Phù thạch: Hòn đá nổi (đá bọt), vị mặn, tính bình không độc, giáng hỏa, trừ đàm, trị mắt mờ, đái gắt, nổi hạch, sưng dái.

486. Đại giả thạch: Hòn son, vị đắng, tính hàn không độc, yên hồn, trừ tà, trừ phong, trị bưng huyết, đau bụng, lở âm hộ.

487. Thạch yến: Yến đá, vị ngọt, tính lành không độc, trị đi tả, đái buốt, bạch trọc, bạch đới, mắt mờ, đẻ khó.

488. Thạch giải: Cua đá, vị mặn, tính hàn, không độc, giải thuốc độc, trị mắt mờ, thanh manh, ung nhọt, bệnh dịch và khó đẻ.

489. Tích lịch châm: Lưỡi tầm sét, tính bình, không độc, trị kinh phong, giết trùng lao, chữa bệnh đái ra cát sỏi và ỉa chảy.

XXI - LOÀI MUỐI KHOÁNG

490. Thực diêm: Muối ăn, vị ngọt, mặn, tính hàn không độc, chữa chứng khí nghịch, tích đờm, đau bụng, giết trùng độc, tiêu phù thũng, sưng lở.

491. Tiêu thạch: Diêm (Diêm tiêu), vị đắng, tính hàn, không độc, chữa bụng đầy trướng, họng tắc, bệnh tích tụ, đái buốt và đau bụng.

492. Bằng sa: Hàn the, vị cay, đắng, tính hơi ấm, không độc, chữa chứng tích cục, đờm đọng, họng đau, nhọt lở và mắt mờ.

493. Lưu hoàng: Sinh (Diêm vàng), vị mặn, mùi hôi tanh, tính ấm, có độc, trị lở loét có trùng, thận lạnh, liệt dương, bổ lao, tổn, chặn cơn kinh giật trẻ con.

XXII - THUỘC VỀ NGƯỜI

494. Loạn phát: Tóc rối. Khi dùng phải đốt ra, vị đắng, tính hơi ấm, không độc, thông quan, cầm máu, chặn cơn kinh trẻ con, chữa các chứng lỵ, lở và đậu mùa (Lược)

495. Trảo giáp: Móng tay, vị ngọt mặn, tính hàn không độc, công dụng khai thông, thúc đẻ, thông đái buốt, cầm máu, chữa chứng phạm phòng và chứng cảm gió. Đốt tồn tính cho uống vào là khỏi ngay.

496. Nhân nha: Răng người, vị ngọt hơi đắng, mặn tính có độc, công dụng chữa sốt rét, nốt đậu bị hãm, lao trùng, nhọt lở và cổ độc.

497. Nhân phấn: Phân người, tính hơi hàn, không độc, thương hàn, sốt nóng phát cuồng mụn độc, nốt đậu bị hãm, bệnh lao nóng âm (đốt ra tro láng nước mà dùng).

498. Đồng tiểu tiện: Nước đái trẻ. Tính hàn không độc, nhuận tim phổi, trừ lao, chặn ho, tiêu máu cục trong bụng, chỉ huyết, sát trùng, thanh nhiệt. Dùng nước đái con trai độ 6, 7 tuổi trở xuống mạnh khỏe là tốt, khi lấy bỏ 4 giọt đầu và 4 giọt cuối đừng dùng.

499. Nhũ trấp: Nước sữa người, vị ngọt, tính mát không độc, bổ khí huyết, chữa hư lao, đau mắt, phong cấm khẩu.

XXIII - NHỮNG VỊ THUỐC LƯỢM LẶT THÊM

(Bản thảo thập dị) gồm 87 vị (15)

1. Bách thiên liệu - Lá đơn tía (lá trên thì xanh, dưới thì tía)
2. Đăng lung thảo - Cây thù lù

15. Phần này do đời sau chép thêm, có một số vị gọi nhầm. Sách in năm 1961 chỉ có 63 vị, sau in lại một lần thêm 19 vị, và lần in năm 1908 lại thêm 5 vị thành 87 vị (bản A.3024). Đây dịch nguyên văn, chú thích của nguyên bản để trong (vòng đơn) đính chính để trong ngoặc vuông.

44

48

recommender systems would prioritize visual over textual content), but also because the overall activity of engaging in photos with one's network represents the ritual of participating in a community built around common interests and ideals (Oeldorf-Hirsch and Sundar, 2016). In engaging with photo-sharing practices on these communities, people not only share photos to talk about images, but also to communicate visually – and phatically, such that the communicative significance of photo sharing lies in the pleasure of the act itself for the sake of visual connectivity (Lobinger, 2016). The coupling of the digital text and the digital image goes deeper than this: images, too, are alphanumeric at the level of storage and processing, and are subject to the same mathematical procedures of signal processing with text.

Figure 4.4 shows a typical post on the *Hội chữa bệnh bằng cây thuốc nam* [Curing diseases with Southern medical plants] Facebook group, where the poster included illustrative photos of the relevant medical plants for herbal recipes to help with stomach and duodenum ulcer, gastroesophageal reflux, and HP bacterial infection. Also included in the post on the left was the original poster's personal contact information (obscured for privacy), offering to sell these cures at a discount price to those going through financial hardship. A sample comment thread to this post has been reproduced on the right. In this comment thread, a group member recalled the story of her neighbour who recently received a stomach cancer diagnosis and could not afford biomedical treatment. Pleading for leads on herbal cures for stomach cancer, the group member described in detail her neighbour's symptoms and suffering – and the neighbour's exemplary morality – in return for much sympathy and compassion from the group. Another group member (shown here) suggested that she looked for other Facebook groups that are centred on sharing Southern medicine cancer cures, with the hope that those going through the same predicament in other discussion groups could offer help.

Even as the anatomy of a Facebook post resembles that of the practical handbook entry, the form of the discussion thread baked into each unit of content on this platform enables not only the dissemination of knowledge as evolution of the printed form, but also as knowledge making and networking. That herbal recipes to help manage gastroesophageal reflux became a site of knowledge making and referencing about stomach cancer is emblematic of the network dynamics explored in Chapter 5 – and of the fundamental distinction between the affordances of the analogue and the digital. The digital text is live; far from being the plain residue of literacy culture, digital text as executable and multivalent is encapsulated in the multi-dimensional grid structure that modulates everything we see – and touch – on the screen. Digital knowledge ecologies are so pliable because their materiality is stratified across intertwined yet incongruent sites, unconstrained by the rigidity of linear mechanisms of analogue inscription. This pliability makes crowdsourcing as a practice possible: if the passing of paper herbal recipes

Figure 4.4: Sample Southern medicine discussion thread on Facebook

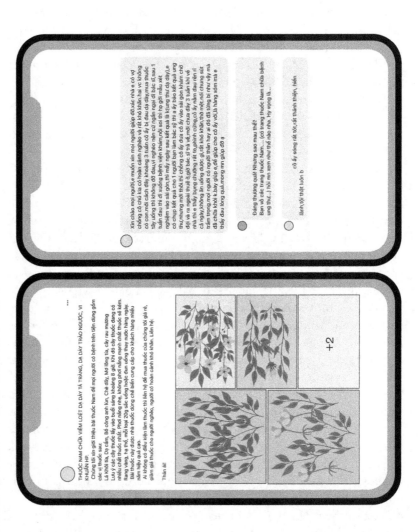

Figure 4.5: Sample Southern medicine discussion comments on Facebook

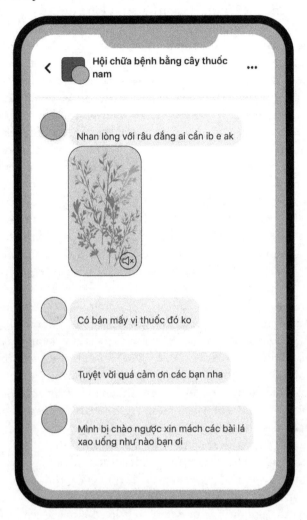

by hand is always subject to error, deterioration, damage, and loss – then the crowd digitization of these recipes on a social media platform such as Facebook not only speeds up and personalizes the process of knowledge propagation, but also enlists these digitized recipes into a new discourse network that gives new permutations not only to their form and content, but also to their sociality (Chapter 5).

Figure 4.5 presents a sample of comments on the same discussion thread in Figure 4.4, where group members variously inquired about where to purchase the relevant ingredients, prompted others to post more recipes to manage stomach pain, expressed gratitude for the information in the post, and – perhaps most interestingly – uploaded raw footage of themselves foraging for Indian pennywort and stinking passionflower, two of the ingredients mentioned in the original post. Using the footage as evidence of provenance, the commenter called for group members to get in touch via private messaging if they were interested in buying these ingredients. The network of digital inscription that can be assembled from these structured and mediated communicative efforts lays bare the socio-collective nature of knowledge production – that which might have stayed hidden in the printed and handwritten forms, following literary conventions where the text as a finished product is never supposed to reveal the process of its making.

The digitization of the written word alongside other media formats means that media no longer store human experience as such; rather, they store the bits of data that 'register molecular increments of behaviour that are never an expression of lived human experience' (Hansen, 2015, p 40). As a result of this, media have shifted from addressing humans first and foremost to registering the environmentality of the world itself, providing a worldly sensibility prior to human consciousness and bodily-based perception (Hansen, 2015). Facebook metrics, such as reacts, comments, and shares, are not the product of indifference of the indices by which the relations are represented. Rather, they are *continually implicated* in an indexical relation to a dynamic environment that is increasingly being operationalized such that what is referred to is not kept separate from or external by the index itself (Lury, 2021). Indexicality and the indices, however, are not indifferent to the objects they index; the network lives of non-biomedical knowledges are not independent of their social lives. Contemporary practices of datafication are associated with transformations in the material-semiotic practices of knowledge-making that can be described as 'bringing the world into the world' (Lury, 2012, quoted in Lury, 2021, p 59). The environment that such a paradigm presupposes can be quantitatively mapped using platform data and the computational methods that underpin their existence, which can helpfully inform our inquiry into the conditions under which lived experiences with digital technologies are possible at all. Chapter 5 uses social network analysis and machine learning techniques to explore a Facebook dataset spanning three different non-biomedical knowledge groups. By using these methods, the chapter explores what automated methods can do to help us uncover the 'hidden' topics within a well-defined dataset under the assumption that these underlying topics match with the probabilistic distribution of words over a set vocabulary – a logic made legible by the digitization of the written word. The chapter also explores the network attributes of these groups, such as whether they exhibit 'small-world' characteristics – and describes the processes of their knowledge propagation using the formal language of network analysis. That this formal language has become routinely applied to the analysis of digital sociality is made possible by ongoing datafication of the media environment – whose lived experience in relation to time and space is explored in Part III.

A note on methods

The previous section presented a mini media archaeology of the written miracle cure from the 18th century until the advent of social media. Media archaeology as method is often discussed in connection with media genealogy, with both approaches relying on Michel Foucault's methodological concepts: his investigations into the archaeology of knowledge (Foucault, 1966) and his history of power in the genealogical sense (Foucault, 1977). Media archaeology is concerned with the material basis of mediality, which tends to freeze the object of its study and view technological shaping of society as ruptures of discrete time layers rather than processes (Ramati and Pinchevski, 2018). Media genealogy, on the other hand, engages ideally with its object – and from the perspective of 'situated knowledge' (Haraway, 1988) that puts an emphasis on continuity and interconnections between historical periods, focusing on mutual influences of society and technologies. The underlying assumption of both methods is that along with technologies, a sort of 'media unconscious' has taken form – the implied knowledge of which can become *visible* with the help of media archaeology (Apprich and Bachmann, 2017). By focusing on points of continuity and rupture in historical processes of media, media archaeology as method offers 'a hermeneutic reading of the "new" against the grain of the past, rather than telling of the histories of technologies from past to present' (Lovink, 2011, p 8). Doing media archaeology means drawing parallels between seemingly incompatible phenomena, constructing histories of suppressed, neglected, and forgotten media that do not point teleologically to the present media-cultural condition, and assembling temporal connections, translations, and mergers between media (Huhtamo and Parikka, 2011). A media archaeology such as that presented in this chapter historicizes the kind of computational analyses done in the next chapter, not only so that we can appreciate the context of their emergence and influence on scholarly inquiry – but also the terms of their utility and limit.

5

Mapping Transnational Networks
of Written Miracles

Miracle cures as online networks

That the digitization of the written word is intimately tied to the digitization of the social was not a coincidence; the internet as technology and social infrastructure is an extremely complicated and multi-faceted system that relies not only on the computing script at the level of executable code, control instructions, and network protocols, but also on natural language input at the level of the user interface. The digitized word coming in from one end is always subject to *post hoc* collection, 'cleaning', transformation, exploration, clustering, classification, regression, and association rule mining – so that they can be made to say useful things about the social processes that are implicated in their inscription. As miracle cures become collectively digitized, the linearity with which they used to be disseminated (from publisher to readers, from medical families to clients, from clients to their extended network of friends and families) become disrupted and diversified. The decentralized and transnational nature of social networking on the internet also scaled up the propagation of miracle cures, thereby increasing the complexity of their multidirectional flows.

Throughout history, knowledges produced by these different social classes received different levels of marginalization under French colonialism and through competition from the more 'learned' and established Chinese medical traditions. *Thuốc Bắc* (Northern medicine), for example, is commonly associated with the literati class and is heavily influenced by Chinese medicine, whereas *thuốc Nam* (Southern medicine) is commonly associated with medical families (Monnais et al, 2011). Those who make a living by scouting, growing, collecting, prescribing, and selling raw medicinal plants also contribute to this knowledge ecosystem with their own interpretations and revisions of family recipes through direct interaction with patients, as well as experience with local flora and fauna.

The propagation of these knowledges throughout history has followed flexible patterns and structures that enabled composition, retention, and reperformance, as well as constant revision. These knowledges fulfil clear and immediate functions for communities that maintain them – namely managing illnesses and preserving health – through their ability to vary and respond to different circumstances. Weak ties among traditional medicine (TM) groups on Facebook, for example, provide various types of social support, including informational, emotional, tangible, esteem, and network support (Nguyen, 2021b). The adoption and domestication of livestreaming technologies on Facebook among emergent non-biomedical therapeutic practices also create alternative temporal spaces for them to thrive at the margin of scientific biomedical practices and at the centre of everyday life (Nguyen, 2021a).

What is not known, however, is whether the democratization of these knowledges through decentralized propagation on social media has changed the very fabric of their sociality: whether new crossovers and contacts are being forged as a result of intensified and increasingly visible flows of these historically marginalized knowledges. Also not well-understood is the content of knowledges being exchanged at the aggregate level, as well as its associated discourses – given the vast volume of data being produced on these sites. What are the network characteristics of Vietnamese non-biomedical sites on Facebook? What types of non-biomedical knowledge discourses are present within these sites? Computational methods developed with the goal of generating data-driven knowledge in the spirit of efficiency, expediency, and privileging the logic of automation – in other words, methods that operate on the mechanical rationality of the digital – can be mobilized towards answering these questions.

Methods

Methodological choices and motivation

This chapter uses social network analysis (SNA) and machine learning techniques (particularly natural language processing and topic modelling) to answer the two research questions. SNA is a set of theoretical perspectives and analytic techniques used to examine how exchanges between individual units shape, and are shaped by, the larger context in which those two individual units are embedded (Carolan, 2016). SNA assumes an emphasis on relations among individuals and not their individual attributes, with a particular focus on individuals not as members of discreet groups, but rather as members of overlapping networks (Marin and Wellman, 2011; Carolan, 2016). Formal network measures provide a rigorous language with which to discern network properties and make sense of the way non-biomedical knowledge propagates on internet environments (Hanneman and Riddle, 2016).

Machine learning techniques, particularly those of an unsupervised nature such as Latent-Dirichlet Allocation (LDA), allow for the statistically driven uncovering of topics 'hidden' in the dataset under the assumption that underlying topics match with the probabilistic distribution of words over a set vocabulary (Blei et al, 2003; Blei and Mcauliffe, 2007). These techniques allow for robust and automated discovery of a large corpus, which is useful for the current context. Subsequent interpretation and labelling of the topics discovered by this automated process are conducted by the researcher, which ensures that these topics are meaningful according to human evaluation standards.

Site selection strategy

The selected sites were purposively sampled from an automated list of 1,900 Vietnamese non-biomedical health groups and pages on Facebook, based on three criteria: (i) popularity, measured in number of active participants; (ii) activity, measured in number of posts per week; and (iii) privacy settings, in that only public sites with fully public content are selected. Criteria (i) and (ii) ensure the sites sampled are active rather than abandoned sites (Hether et al, 2016; Smith and Graham, 2019). Criterion (iii) ensures that automatic collection of textual data does not violate participants' privacy; informed consent was not sought because participants were engaged in a public discussion and no personally identifiable information was collected. These criteria are also consistent with what van Dijck and Poell (2013) theorize as the four grounding principles of social media logic: programmability (the mutual layering of technological features and human agency in shaping platform usage); popularity (the algorithmic and socioeconomic conditioning of influence and importance); connectivity (socio-technical affordances of the platform apparatus that mediate user activity); and datafication (the ability of network platforms to render into data aspects of life that were not quantified before). Only sites with over 30,000 members and a posting frequency of over ten posts per day were selected for the sample. The automated list was generated by automating searches using the search function on Facebook with 21 different keywords. Table 5.1 provides descriptive statistics of the sampled sites.

Facebook has been chosen as the platform in focus, despite changes to the Graph API in 2016 following the Cambridge Analytica scandal (Albright, 2018), as it remains the most popular social network site in the world and the fastest growing platform in Vietnam and South East Asia (Kemp, 2023). Facebook is the most popular social network site in Vietnam; Vietnam is Facebook's seventh-largest market worldwide (Kemp, 2023; We Are Social, 2023).

The sites sampled here are public sites where membership is not moderated, as opposed to moderated membership where applicants are required to answer

Table 5.1: Descriptive statistics of sampled sites (as of August 2019)

Site	Number of members	Number of posts	Number of comments	Number of 'reacts'	Number of 'shares'
Site 1 Good traditional medical recipes (*Các bài thuốc dân gian hay*)	38,744	3,940	16,459	55,511	13,921
Site 2 Southern medicinal plants and family recipes (*Cây thuốc nam và những bài thuốc gia truyền*)	82,008	2,983	6,874	36,159	69,120
Site 3 Your wise medical cabinet (*Tủ thuốc thông thái*)	45,829	1,034	17,699	94	29
Total	166,581	7,957	41,032	91,764	83,070

a set of questions to gain access approval from site administrators. As such, gatekeeping within these sites is minimal. Sites 1 and 2 are more similar to each other than they are to Site 3 in that they are both built exclusively around promoting and sharing Vietnamese traditional medical recipes. Site 1 centres on the sharing of traditional Vietnamese medicine in general, while Site 2 is focused on Southern medicine and family recipes. Site 3 has an explicit anti-biomedicine philosophy; the site description outlines its advocacy against over-reliance on biomedicine as an expensive therapeutic option. Each of these sites corresponds to a different existing knowledge paradigm that characterizes the diversity of non-biomedical practices in Vietnam. Together, these sites are the top active sites for the exchange of non-biomedical knowledge on Facebook in Vietnam.

Data collection and network generation

Data were collected with a purpose-built web scraper. The scraper utilizes the Puppeteer library developed by Google to collect publicly available data via the Chrome web browser. The scraper collected all text content on original posts and their associated comments over five years, from 19 August 2014 to 19 August 2019. As shown in Table 5.1, the dataset contains 7,957 unique posts and 41,032 comments, representing the activities of 166,581 unique members. Table 5.1 also includes the total number of 'shares' across all posts for each of the three public sites. A 'share' means that a viewer of a post has shared the post and any associated links within their personal network. All

Table 5.2: Descriptive statistics for constructed co-commenting networks

Site	Nodes	Edges	Density
1	3,560	10,208	0.000805
2	2,783	5,136	0.000663
3	5,475	12,137	0.000405

together for this dataset, posts were shared over 80,000 times. A 'react' on Facebook is an emotional response that takes on one out of six available emotional reactions, signified by six distinct emojis. Due to the limits of non-API scraping, finer data for the 'react' construct are not available. There were altogether 91,764 reacts in this dataset. Although site 3 has a significant number of members and a high count of commenting activity, their 'React' and 'Share' metrics are significantly lower than sites 1 and 2. This peculiar dynamic could be due to the nature of site 3 as a consumer movement site; while the positive framing of knowledge propagation found in sites 1 and 2 might entice more affective engagement and sharing behaviour, the negative framing of site 3 (anti-biomedicine) might limit these forms of engagement. Table 5.2 provides descriptive statistics for the co-commenting networks constructed from the data collected, with density measuring the prevalence of dyadic linkage or direct tie within a social network (Frey, 2018). The index of network density is expressed as the ratio of observed ties (edges) to all possible pairwise ties in a network, whose value ranges between 0 and 1. It can be interpreted as the proportion of potential ties that are actually present (Frey, 2018).

Results

Network analysis

From the data collected, undirected co-commenting activity networks were constructed for each site, wherein nodes represent unique users and edges represent comments. An undirected edge is created if users co-commented on any posts; a low bar is therefore set for creating a relationship between users (Smith and Graham, 2019). Two users are connected if they have both commented on the same post within the five-year time period. This construction adapted the methods proposed by Graham and Ackland (2016), as data on 'Reacts' and 'Shares' could not be collected with the current non-API scraper. Figure 5.1 illustrates the structure of the networks constructed, wherein the thickness of the edges represents the weight value associated with the frequency of co-commenting between users.

User comment networks provide a more fine-grained understanding of the structure and nature of user interactivity on Vietnamese non-biomedical

Figure 5.1: Structure of the constructed Facebook co-commenting activity network

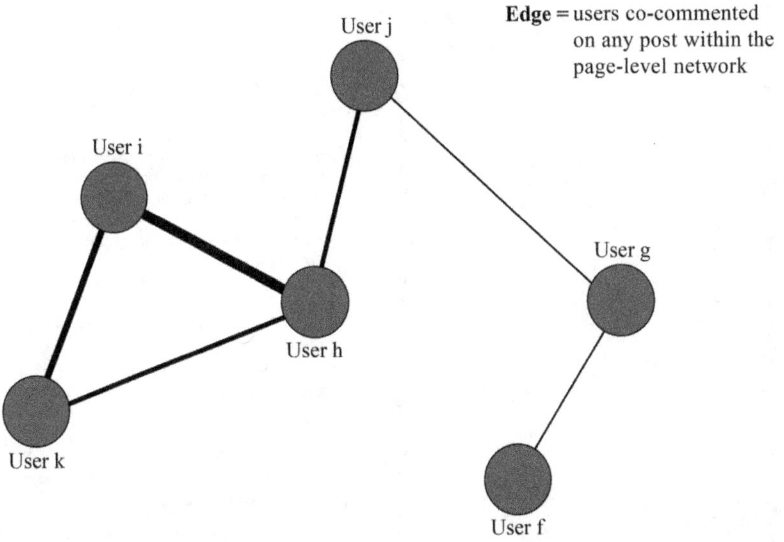

Source: Adapted from Smith and Graham (2019)

knowledge sites, even though Facebook does not directly provide this type of data. Comments are individually composed as open-text and as such represent a novel contribution and extension to discussion, as compared to a reproduction of a previous contribution through reacting or sharing. Comments also contribute differently to the propagation of non-biomedical knowledge on Facebook, as users often read one another's comments, interpret and learn from them, as well as engage in discourse by posting their own comments (Smith and Graham, 2019). Within online health contexts, users actively seek and provide various types of social support through interacting with one another via the interface of social media platforms (Hether et al, 2016; Nguyen, 2021a). As such, these networks provide interesting insights into user (co-)participation and discourse dynamics not only within each site, but also across these sites as an aggregate network. Figure 5.2 presents a sample discussion thread from the dataset.

Although a large number of users are members of these sites, only a small portion of users participated in the form of commenting regularly. As Table 5.3 shows, a majority of users only commented on a post once or twice over a five-year period, which constitutes a highly skewed out-degree distribution. Only a small subset of users within each site contributes in terms of posting content and commenting frequently, and there is a 'long tail' of users who are very infrequent in their commenting activity. This finding is similar to what Smith and Graham (2019) found in their study of anti-vaccination Facebook groups in Australia – where 'transient users', whose

Figure 5.2: Sample Facebook thread from the dataset (usernames are hidden)

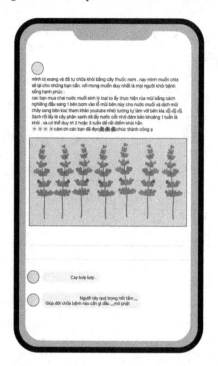

Text translation:

Post content: "I used to have sinusitis and I had it cured by southern medicine plants. Now I want to share to anyone that needs it. My only hope is that everyone will no longer be sick and be happy: Buy a big bottle of saline solution then perform nose washing by tilting your head to one side. Pumping the solution into one nostril until the solution and nasal fluid flow to the other one (please also consult Youtube) then do the same with the other nostril ✿✿✿. Once it's clean, pound the green manure leaves to get its extract and pump it into your nose. I guarantee it will be gone after around one week. And you can maintain for two to three weeks for it to be completely gone. ✿✿✿✿ Thanks for reading ✿✿✿ Good luck.";

Comment 1: "But this is Siam weed";
Comment 2: "This person is a treasure... They are giving medical help without asking for anything return... Namo amitabud.")

Table 5.3: Out-degree distribution of user activity by site-level network

Network	Number of users who commented twice or less	Percentage of total activity within network
Site 1	2,082	55.24
Site 2	1,606	54.66
Site 3	3,904	70.64

participation in anti-vaccination Facebook sites is few and far between – also dominated their sample. This could be indicative of larger trends in user participation on Facebook within health-related groups across different contexts, although further research is needed to examine these dynamics. On an aggregate network level, it is of interest to examine whether users who participate in one site-level network also participate in other sites within the sample. Perhaps quite surprisingly, the percentage of cross-participation within the selected sites is very low (see Table 5.4). In each pair of the site-level network, cross-participation is below 1 per cent, with a particularly low cross-participation rate between sites 2 and 3. As such, not only does site 3 have a very low affective engagement rate ('Reacts') and sharing behaviour

Table 5.4: Percentage of user participation across pairs of site-level networks

	Site 1	Site 2	Site 3
Site 1	100%	0.83%	0.46%
Site 2	0.83%	100%	0.06%
Site 3	0.46%	0.06%	100%

within the site itself, its members also do not seem to engage in the other most popular non-biomedical knowledge sites. Contrasting this against the high intensity of discussion that happens within the site (high counts of comments and posts), it seems that non-biomedical knowledge groups that rely on an anti-biomedicine philosophy could be exhibiting cult-like behaviour, in the sense that content is frequently discussed within, but does not propagate outside of, the group. This implies a sense of insularity that does not benefit knowledge exchange among the examined groups. However, overall low cross-participation rates across the sampled sites are again consistent with what Smith and Graham (2019) have found in their anti-vaccination study. This further supports the observation of the 'transient user' on Facebook, wherein users 'pass by' discursive groups without investing in maintaining discursive relationships or coordinating different discourses across groups.

Considering that each network from the sampled sites remains largely separate from one another, it is worthwhile to further examine whether these networks exhibit the properties of 'small world' networks (Watts and Strogatz, 1998). Small world networks are network structures that are both highly locally clustered and have a short path length – two network characteristics that are usually divergent (Watts, 1999). Small world networks are interesting for many reasons. For example, small world networks enable infectious diseases to spread much more quickly and easily than other types of networks, as the dynamics of the network is an 'explicit function of structure' (Watts and Strogatz, 1998, p 441). Empirical research has also shown that the more a network exhibits characteristics of a small world, the more connected actors are to one another and connected by persons who know one another well through past interactions, or through having had past interactions with common third parties (Uzzi and Spiro, 2005). These conditions allow information circulated in separate clusters to also circulate to other clusters, and to gain the credibility that unfamiliar materials require to be regarded as valuable in new contexts and subsequently used by other members of other clusters (Uzzi and Spiro, 2005). Small world networks are also interesting because they are robust and resistant to damage, in the sense that randomly removing nodes from the network will not significantly impact the effectiveness and dynamics of the network (Smith and Graham, 2019).

The small world phenomenon is not only common in sparse networks with many vertices, as even a tiny fraction of short cuts would suffice. Research has demonstrated that it is also common in biological, social, and artificial systems (Watts and Strogatz,1998; Uzzi et al, 2007; Telesford et al, 2011; Bassett et al, 2017; Opsahl et al, 2017; Smith and Graham, 2019).

Two methods were used to assess whether the three co-commenting networks are 'small worlds'. The first approach follows the conditions set in Watts and Strogatz (1998), where a network is considered small world if (1) its average local clustering coefficient is much greater than a random network generated from the same set of vertices and (2) the mean shortest path length of the network is approximately the same as the associated random network. To do this, I calculated the average local clustering coefficient and mean shortest path length for the three networks studied here and compared these metrics against those of three randomly generated networks with the same number of edge sets. I generated these three random networks using the Erdős-Rényi model implementation in the 'igraph' R package (Csardi and Nepusz, 2006). The second approach employs Humphries and Gurney's (2008) small-worldness index, where the index is calculated as transitivity (normalized by the random transitivity) over the average shortest path length (normalized by the random average shortest path length). Transitivity, an alternative definition of network clustering, is understood as the propensity for two neighbours of a network node also to be neighbours of each other (Newman et al, 2000; Newman, 2009). Using the 'qgraph' R package (Epskamp et al, 2019), the average of the same indices was calculated on 1,000 random networks for each co-commenting network. A network can be said to be 'small world' if its small world index is higher than 1; a stricter rule requires the index to be higher than 3 (Humphries and Gurney, 2008). Results are presented in Table 5.5, where all three networks satisfy the conditions in both approaches to be small worlds.

Text analysis and topic modelling

In order to understand the nature of discourse on these networks, topic modelling was performed on the complete set of textual data collected, including original posts and their associated comments, across all three sites. Probabilistic topic modelling allows for efficient and reproducible analysis of large amounts of textual data without requiring prior annotations or labelling of the textual corpus; topics that emerge from this analysis are determined through the co-occurrence of words and the themes they carry within the texts (Blei, 2012). The analysis was carried out using the LDA method (Blei et al, 2003; Blei and Mcauliffe, 2007), an established generative statistical topic modelling method within the social sciences (DiMaggio, 2015). LDA defines a topic as a distribution over a fixed vocabulary; it assumes that topics

Table 5.5: 'Small world' metrics for user co-comment networks vs random graphs (bolded in brackets) and small-worldness index

Network	Average local clustering coefficient	Average shortest path length	Small-worldness index
Site 1	0.0214 **(0.0018)**	4.414 **(4.871)**	3.353
Site 2	0.0058 **(0.0014)**	5.525 **(6.152)**	9.689
Site 3	0.0099 **(0.0007)**	4.316 **(5.933)**	9.704

Source: Humphries and Gurney (2008)

are specified before textual data are generated (Blei, 2012). This method formalizes the intuition that there exist hidden topics within set texts, and that these hidden topics can be inferred through examining words that appear with particular probabilities. The utility of topic models lies in the property that the hidden structures inferred resemble the thematic structure of the dataset (Blei, 2012).

To prepare the corpus for LDA, a natural language processing annotation pipeline specific to the Vietnamese language was used to segment individual words and tag them with the appropriate part-of-speech (Vu et al, 2018). The analysis was then conducted on 469,388 noun terms, such as 'cancer', 'monk fruit', and 'hibiscus', which occur in at least 80 per cent of 25,356 discussion threads in the dataset. The rationale behind this method is based on the observation that, within this dataset, discussions usually involve support-seeking and provision (that is, people naming a disease or condition to seek out names of medicinal plants or ingredients that supposedly help with said disease or condition). As such, disease names and names of medicinal plants or ingredients that appear alongside each other in the same discussion threads with high frequency could indicate popular non-biomedical therapeutic beliefs and practices. Specifying the LDA model consists of three steps: (i) draw k topics from a symmetric Dirichlet distribution; (ii) for each document d, draw topic proportions from a symmetric Dirichlet distribution; and (iii) for each word n in each document d, draw a topic assignment from the topic proportions and draw the word from a multinomial probability distribution conditioned on the topic (Grün and Hornik, 2011). There are many approaches to choosing k number of topics, such as perplexity (Blei et al, 2003), marginal likelihood (Griffiths and Steyvers, 2004), density (Cao et al, 2009), and symmetric Kullback–Leibler divergence (Arun et al, 2010). No one approach is currently considered the standard; researchers working with LDA often choose the method most appropriate with the nature of their data (Smith and Graham, 2019). To ensure rigorous k selection, I calculated all four metrics using the 'ldatuning' and 'topicmodels' R packages (Grün

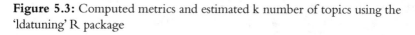

Figure 5.3: Computed metrics and estimated k number of topics using the 'ldatuning' R package

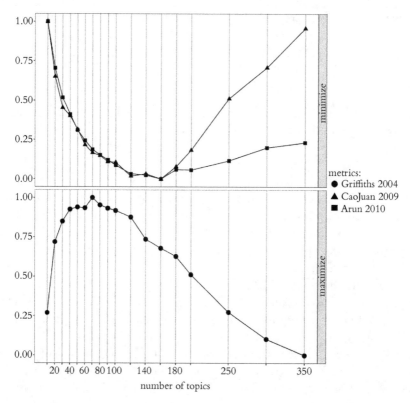

and Hornik, 2011; Nikita, 2016). Figures 5.3 and 5.4 plot the results of these metrics. Figure 5.3 indicates that the best number of topics lies somewhere in the range between 70 and 160, while Figure 5.4 indicates that the range is between 60 and 80. It is documented that Cao et al (2009) and Arun et al (2010) metrics tend to overfit the data (Gerlach et al, 2018; Hou-Liu, 2018). Marginal likelihood (Griffiths and Steyvers, 2004) has been widely used as a measure to specify k on large-scale social media datasets across different languages and health topics, where the topic candidate with the highest likelihood value is considered the best fit (Paul and Dredze, 2012; Ma et al, 2016; Liebeskind & Liebeskind, 2018; Zhao, 2018; Ríssola et al, 2019). Perplexity is often used alongside marginal likelihood as a method of cross-validating k selection, where lower perplexity is considered better fit (Hoang, 2015). Based on these analyses, k topic is selected at 70.

To validate the topic model fitted to the current data, Maier et al (2018) suggested employing 'systematically structured combinations of existing metrics and in-depth investigation to boost the significance of the

Figure 5.4: Computed perplexity and estimated k number of topics using the 'topicmodel' R package

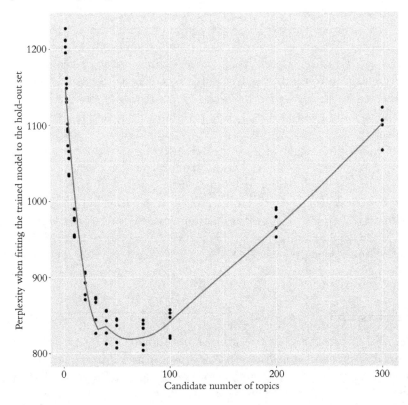

validation process' (p 97). They devised a three-step process to operationalize this: summarizing the most important quantitative information from the model, outlining exclusion strategies for uninterpretable topics, and close reading of the data and labelling of topic.

Maier et al (2018) proposed the use of four particular metrics: rank-1 metric (Evans, 2014), coherence (Mimno et al, 2011), relevance (Sievert and Shirley, 2014), and the Hirschman-Herfindahl Index (HHI). Rank-1 metric is useful for helping identify background topics. Coherence score, when applied to single topics, can help guide intuition in interpretation. Relevance score can help reorder the top words of a topic by considering their overall corpus frequency through manipulating the weighting parameter λ, with best interpretability of topics using a λ-value close to 0.6 (Sievert and Shirley, 2014). Finally, HHI = 1 signifies maximum concentration (the topic is pronounced by only one source) and a very low HHI value, conversely, indicates that a topic can be found in many sources. HHI, while useful in Maier et al's (2018) specific dataset which tracks the hyperlink network of over 300,000 websites, is not useful to the current Facebook dataset. HHI is therefore not calculated here. A sample summary statistics of these metrics is included in Appendix 2.

Of the 70 topics generated, there were 17 overlapping topics (that is, topic 2 appearing 17 times in the results). Only four topics include mostly 'junk' terms such as 'shhh', 'kkkkk', 'hehehehe' – which are words that were not interpretable in relation to others in the topic. These terms are generally considered to be an artifact of social media data and the phatic nature of online communication, which is commonly encountered (Smith and Graham, 2019). These four topics, which contain mostly 'junk terms', are also excluded from analysis. From this filtering process, there are 49 topics that are eligible for analysis. The most representative threads containing each identified topic were retrieved; a close reading of each thread was then conducted manually to ensure that the topic labelling is reflective of the underlying topic by human evaluation standard. This is an indispensable step as the labelling of topics should be constructed on the basis of broader context knowledge (Maier et al, 2018). The final analysis of the remaining 49 topics is presented in Appendix 1, Table A.1, together with relevant statistics.

Discussion

The analysis presented in this chapter has shown that Vietnamese non-biomedical networks on Facebook are quite sparse: they do not seem to function as close-knit communities of knowledge exchange and support, where participants interact in a sustained fashion over time. The nature of this social exchange pattern diverges from how traditional medical knowledge has historically been passed down from generation to generation in Vietnam, which relied on upholding, and sometimes gatekeeping, closed therapy communities. This does not mean, however, that traditional medical knowledge is being 'democratized' as such. There is very little cross-pollination of knowledge sharing among the three sampled sites; people who participate in one site are not likely to also participate in others. Considering that each of these sites was organized around a different therapeutic regime (Southern medicine vs 'traditional' Northern medicine) with different philosophical outlooks (consumer advocacy vs agenda-free knowledge sharing), the analysis seems to be suggesting that existing boundaries among different 'traditions' are being replicated online. This pattern is similar to the behaviour of, for example, Australian anti-vaccination pages on Facebook, where cross-group participation is also not prevalent (Smith and Graham, 2019). More research examining this emerging dynamic of Facebook groups and pages is warranted, especially against the context of Facebook redesigning its interface to prioritize interest-based group and community interactions to mitigate uses of the platform merely as an 'address book' (Statt, 2019).

The lack of coordination across these sites might also have deeper roots in existing social mechanisms that maintain the propagation of traditional medical knowledge. Craig (2002) noted how the legacy of Vietnamese family health knowledge and practice, transmitted in its most durable forms through oral traditions and written recipes, is located within the household level where it is readily put to use. Since this locates the primary caregiving responsibility within the family unit rather than with professionals and institutions or online strangers, the logic that drives the propagation of non-biomedical knowledge is that of use-value: that people seek traditional medical knowledges in times of sickness and share them mostly in response to those in need in a transactional fashion. Unsolicited sharing of recipes and knowledges, when it happens, also seems to be grounded in collectively imagined boundaries between various undercurrents of TM. The lack of cross-pollination among different 'traditions' and consumer movements – Southern medicine vs Northern medicine vs Anti-biomedicine – seems to be replicating itself online, where people engage in rather insular and separate networks that map onto existing knowledge paradigms that are anchored in well-established everyday practices.

Despite the lack of interaction across different sites, network activities within the sites themselves are quite robust and resistant to change. All three networks exhibit 'small world' characteristics – which structurally enables quick and easy propagation of information. It is in this regard that Vietnamese non-biomedical networks resemble the characteristics of other networks on Facebook (Catanese et al, 2011; Caci et al, 2012; Wohlgemuth and Matache, 2012; Smith and Graham, 2019). This analysis contributes to the growing body of evidence of the ubiquity of small-world networks on Facebook, which could indicate that the affordances of Facebook as a platform might be shaping networks towards 'small-worldness'. If this is the case, then the growing popularity of self-contained community groups on Facebook might be fertile ground for resilient and durable discourse communities. Future research should look at the new temporalities that this mediated sociality is giving to the information and knowledge being propagated on social networking sites such as Facebook, especially with regard to rich and complex multimedia formats such as livestreaming videos and synchronous viewing of pre-recorded videos.

Following the Latourian approach to tracing the interactions and discourses left behind by actors in this knowledge network also means acknowledging the co-production of sociality and materiality (Latour, 2005; Law and Mol, 1995). Materials are relational effects; when we look at the social, we are also looking at the production of materiality. This materiality need not stop at the collection of texts exchanged, photos shared, videos uploaded, or livestreams watched; the material heterogeneity of networks extends to people, medicines, money, institutions, food, and TM clinics. Artifacts of this sort could embody social relations in materials more durable than those in online interactions. Durability is a relational effect; the strategies that reside within the materiality and affordances of things are contingent on durability as much as the manipulability and scale of these materials. A recipe shared as text on Facebook has a different malleability and tractability to a video instructing how to follow the same recipe, or suggestions on where to buy the necessary ingredients, or offers to send these ingredients through the mail to those who want them. Strategies or strategic loci of things are recursive and reflexive effects produced in a space where materials of different durability and manipulability join together (Law and Mol, 1995). Following this, the discourse network traced here is not the end, but rather the beginning of reassembling the actor-network anew by the passage of another medium, another circulating entity (Michael, 2017). The computational analyses conducted in this chapter, while not addressing the materialistic conditions of the texts collected, serve as a reminder about the materiality that is already embedded in networks beyond the visible traces of data that can readily be collected as a result of platform enclosure of human behaviour (Wu and Taneja, 2021).

Some cues as to how to continue this tracing can be found by looking into the discourse content existing within the networks traced. With the LDA method, 49 unique topics were identified and qualitatively labelled. The significant number of overlapping topics found within the dataset is reflective of both the nature of social networking behaviour and the way in which TM is communicated in Vietnamese. Reposting popular and interesting content found elsewhere is common behaviour on social media (Lu et al, 2014; Wang et al, 2019a), making frequently recurring content characteristic to social media data. LDA modelling picked up this pattern in the dataset.

Overall, the topics identified through LDA can fit under eight broad themes: managing health and illnesses (topics 2–12, 14–17, 19–20, 24–5, 28–33, 35–40, 45–9), institutionalization of TM (topic 1), origins and legitimacy (topic 23), sales (topics 3, 7, 26, 27), lifestyle (topics 6, 21, 22, 34), religion and philanthropy (topic 4), negative aspects to TM (topics 13, 18, 42), and TM and overseas Vietnamese (topics 14, 16, 44). Among these broad themes, the last three themes are probably the most interesting. A close reading of posts containing the theme of religion and philanthropy reveals that Buddhist temples remain an important locus through which people of disadvantaged socioeconomic background in Vietnam seek and receive health care. TM, usually in the form of raw ingredients, is also frequently distributed for free by monks who practise medicine through Buddhist temples. This is an interesting finding, as it is pointing to the informal yet significant health-care role that religious institutions continue to play, especially in a secular, post-socialist society such as Vietnam. As we have seen in the previous chapters, one of the earliest extant Vietnamese medical texts, 'Miraculous Drugs of the South' (*Nam Dược Thần Hiệu*), was written by the Vietnamese Buddhist monk-physician *Tuệ Tĩnh*. For many centuries in Vietnam and East and South East Asia more generally, it was common for Buddhist monks and nuns to work as healers; Buddhist contexts have continued to be the most important loci for the cross-cultural exchange of diverse currents of medicine ideas and practices concerning illness and healing (Thompson, 2017b). Local traditions of Buddhist medicine represent unique hybrid combinations of cross-culturally transmitted and indigenous knowledge (Salguero, 2018). In addition to the transformations happening to Buddhist medicine by means of interactions with Western colonialism, scientific ideas, and new biomedical technologies, the internet and its social media platforms are the latest actors to contribute to the evolution and persistence of these non-biomedical modalities.

Critical discussions against TM are also present on these networks. There appear to be negotiations of what constitutes legitimate uses of medicinal plants, and indeed what counts as 'medicine' through these critical discussions. For example, in one discussion, speculations on the medicinal properties of shrimp paste – a South East Asian fermented condiment – were criticized as nonsensical and labelled as 'country bumpkin' thinking. 'Food as medicine' has long been a prominent characteristic in the East and South East Asian systems of medical thought, where local food cultures are inseparable from traditional therapeutic systems (Ogle et al, 2003; Pieroni and Price, 2006). The perceived multiple functions of edible plants and local food, however, are not immutable; as the above example shows, the medicinal functions of local food are subject to ongoing negotiation and reinterpretations as understandings about nutrition and health evolve. Future research could look into the ways in which living discourses surrounding policing and adjudicating the boundaries between food and medicine intersect with processes of urbanization and modernization, as well as how the changing distinction between functional foods and food medicines is being played out on social media.

Finally, it appears that the discourses conducted on and through these sites are transnational in nature. *Việt Kiều*, or overseas Vietnamese, are present in these online discussions; they are distinct actors insofar as they facilitate discussion topics that are distinct from those who reside inside Vietnam. These discussions involve, among others, requests for and provision of referrals to unlicensed traditional medical practices outside of Vietnam, and transnational trading of herbal ingredients through informal means. It is estimated that there are around 4.5 million Vietnamese living overseas, contributing USD15.9 billion to the Vietnamese economy annually in remittances (Minh Huy, 2018). The majority of the Vietnamese diaspora left Vietnam as political and economic refugees at the end of the Vietnam War in 1975; almost half of overseas Vietnamese reside in the United States, and the majority of *Việt Kiều* live in other industrialized countries such as Japan, France, Australia, and Canada. Given that non-biomedical therapies are much more marginalized and stigmatized in these societies, future research could look at the ways in which diasporic communities navigate, with or without success, the health-care systems of host-states while forging and maintaining links with the 'homeland' through participating in networked propagation of traditional knowledges. Beyond issues concerning the navigation of biomedical health systems, issues with transnational belonging and emergent hybrid narratives about health and illness may also manifest themselves in novel ways through these networks. Furthermore, these network connections have the potential to materialize through the increasingly dense networks of transnational mobility.

Many of the discussions involving overseas Vietnamese also involved word-of-mouth referrals to private non-biomedical practices both within and outside of Vietnam, sales of medicinal plants and deliberations of international shipment details, and negotiations of international money transfers – through both formal and informal channels. The ways in which online networks manifest themselves materially beyond digitally enabled interactions, particularly in health contexts, warrant closer attention in future studies. It is important to note that although material and social relations might be matters of local performance, they may not 'add up' to form an overall pattern or structure (Latour, 2005; Law and Mol, 1995). This 'patchwork' outlook, while promising to neither tell coherent stories nor provide a complete map of actors and their connections, is faithful to material multiplicity and committed to the generalized symmetry that treats material differences not as given, but rather generated in relations themselves.

Conclusion

This chapter explored the network dynamics of, and discourses present within, Vietnamese non-biomedical discussion sites on Facebook. By combining natural language processing and generative topic modelling techniques to explore a large-scale online dataset in the Vietnamese language, this chapter explores the proverbial network life of traditional medical knowledges on the internet. While limited by the sites sampled, the analysis presented here provides a foundational and empirically driven account of online propagation of traditional knowledges. The goal was not to exhaust all possible social media content, but rather to provide a rigorous analysis and suggest future directions in an under-researched topic that could have important implications in different disciplines. Vietnamese non-biomedical knowledges are propagating on social media with mechanisms that seem to be replicating existing socially and culturally constrained boundaries of knowledge regimes, with little evidence of cross-pollination between different 'traditions' of knowledge. The open and transnational nature of social media, however, has allowed for micro (national religion and philanthropy, negotiations of meaning and legitimacy) and macro (diasporic networks of resource and care) processes to unfold with increasing visibility and reach.

The social-network lives of non-biomedical knowledge, as such, are distributed rather than contained; they do not reside within imagined boundaries of platforms, but traverse across many places at a time, and many times at one place. The problem with 'platform seeing', where seeing is a position from a singular mode of observation, is that many visual elements, techniques, and forms of observing are highly distributed through data practices of collection, analysis, and prediction (Mackenzie and Munster, 2019). Formal analyses of platform data such as the kind done in this chapter tell only part of the story. What I am interested in in Part III is to examine the lived experiences of people who rely on non-biomedical knowledge and practices for their survival – be it in their professional practice of these modalities as the primary mode of income, or in their engagement with these modalities as a tactic of managing the experiences of illness of their own and their loved ones. In the coming pages, I explore the activities and stories that leave no discernible trace on social media platforms, yet happen alongside these traces. These activities and stories give broader context to the digital traces they accompany and, when put together, they give us a richer understanding of the social lives of digital miracle cures.

PART III

Digital Miracles as Digital Play

Prologue: Embodying the digital

Our bodily activities are increasingly directly connected to the use of technological devices, as we carry our laptops, phones, and other electronic items throughout the day: we rely on these devices to communicate, socialize, stay productive, and, as we will see in the following chapters, enact miracles. We no longer use digital technologies simply to communicate, as the previous section has dissected; as we engage with these technologies beyond textual modes, our bodily performance in the digital milieu becomes richly entwined in the dynamic technological affordances that are already embedded in distinct cultural contexts and collective habits. What does it mean to perform digital miracles? What are the sociotechnical conditions that make digital miracles possible?

The ease with which digital images can be produced with digital devices has transformed the social mode of photography and videography from a fixed position of being gazed at and consumed to a dynamic visual practice that is intended to be shared, discussed, and revisited. This transformation not only changes the language of vernacular image-making, but also the very conditions of possibility of creative, spiritual, and miraculous pursuits. Because taking photos and videos has become routine and mundane practice thanks to increasingly ubiquitous availability of devices and internet access, it is to the level of the everyday that we should now turn our attention. In this section, we will interrogate the conditions of possibility for living with digital miracles through a complex digital mode of engagement: that of platform livestreaming.

6

If It's Worth Doing, It's Worth Doing Live: Livestreaming Miracles

What kind of time do we experience when we wait? When we wait for someone to turn up to a video call, time feels like an interlude; when we wait for our Facebook News Feed to load, time feels like a clot in our throat as the buffering icon keeps on spinning. In waiting, we realize that there is a multitude to temporalities: time can be standardized so people can be in the same place at the same time, but time also dwells inside each of us – in the consciousness of our finite lifetime and in the rhythms of our body. Technology has been said to accelerate time and contract duration (Hassan, 2011; Wajcman, 2015); what, then, of waiting with technology? Technology has not made waiting redundant, but it seems to have transformed waiting substantially. When we reach for our phone as we wait, with or without a direction, waiting is given shape outside of our own body. When we wait on or with our phone, however, waiting re-emerges as viscerally within.

Liveness captures some of these entangled dynamics of waiting in the presence of technology. Certain temporal arrangements are to be made for liveness to be enacted: someone to 'go live', someone to 'watch live', something to be happening 'live', some technologies to faithfully carry out 'the live'. Radio is thought of as a live medium (Vianello, 1985), broadcast television is live insofar as it competes with the new viewing platforms and business models such as Netflix and Hulu (van Es, 2017), 'digital liveness' has been understood as 'our conscious act of grasping virtual entities as live in response to the claims they make on us' (Auslander, 2012, p 10). Liveness temporality is multiple and contingent on its medium; the 'paradox of liveness' lies in its apparent constructedness and its seeming claim to provide direct access to the event relayed (van Es, 2017). There is a similar paradox to the temporality of waiting: waiting is an enactment of particular bodily and extra-bodily temporalities, but waiting is also time temporalizing through the body.

In the sections that follow, I explore what it means when people engage in liveness as a way to overcome waiting – to recalibrate downtime. I begin by outlining the paradox of liveness as algorithmic and liveness as lived by reviewing current disparate literatures. I proceed by establishing the relationship between liveness and time in the presence of technology through a discussion of 'medial *eigenzeit*'. I have chosen the mediatized practice of *diện chẩn* – a Vietnamese unregulated therapeutic method – on Facebook Live as the case study. In my discussion of this case, I reflect on my fieldwork in the US and Vietnam where I interviewed and observed the practices of *diện chẩn* livestreamers and audiences over a period of two years. While the case examined here is local and particular, I hope to show that the reverberation of downtime and liveness temporalities has created an alternative temporal space for practices whose temporality is at odds with the temporal structure of institutions and society. Furthermore, it is through my discussion of the case that I develop my conceptualization of downtime as multiscale: downtime exists in between the micro action and inaction of everyday life, but also in larger episodes of personal and health crises that reorient the body towards technologies for instantaneous replenishment of meaning and activity. Viewing liveness through the analytical lens of downtime allows us to trace the mechanisms in which liveness is variously enacted as a particular interaction between institutions, technologies, and people. It also allows us to trace the emergence of tactical digital temporal spaces that thrive at the margin of more enduring institutional temporal structures.

The apparent paradox of Facebook Live

Since Facebook publicly launched its social livestreaming service Facebook Live in 2016, the platform has vigorously pushed the service through its technical and commercial infrastructure, going as far as tweaking its algorithm to favour live videos (Rein and Venturini, 2018). In a post that commemorates the launch of this service on 6 April 2016, Mark Zuckerberg said:

> Live is like having a TV camera in your pocket. Anyone with a phone now has the power to broadcast to anyone in the world. When you interact live, you feel connected in a more personal way. This is a big shift in how we communicate, and it's going to create new opportunities for people to come together. (Zuckerberg, 2016)

Facebook Live was developed with an amalgamation of the 'media logic' that permeates the imagination of Silicon Valley: individual communication power, 24/7 content broadcast, user interactivity, and unsubstantiated connectedness. While applications for real-time video transmission over the internet are not new, live video as a social medium is a more recent phenomenon, with earliest social livestreaming platforms such as ComVu Pocket Caster launched in 2005, followed by Bambuser and Ustream (Juhlin et al, 2010). Facebook Live as one of the latest additions to the Facebook ecosystem not only inherits and innovates against the technologies that came before, but also actively shapes the evolution of video livestreaming as a major influence. Rein and Venturini (2018) showed how, through strategic partnership and technological infrastructural tweaks, Facebook Live is far from a case of 'spontaneous innovation'. Instead, Facebook Live influences both the editorial organization as well as the storytelling of live video streaming, co-producing rather than simply facilitating livestreaming content. This co-production ushers in temporalities specific to the artificial figuration of Facebook Live as an assemblage – the evolving arrangement of which co-emerges with specific user subjectivities that would then feed back into this arrangement. In 2017, one out of five videos on Facebook was a live broadcast; Facebook Live videos produce six times as many interactions as traditional videos and 165 per cent more comments than on-demand videos, and retain the attention of users three times as long (99firms, 2023).

In a computationally extensive study, Raman et al (2018) analyzed 3TB of Facebook Live data for patterns of global activity only to question whether the platform is 'truly' live, or indeed can even be considered a 'broadcast' service at all. This conclusion is drawn from the findings that, despite gathering much more engagement compared to traditional non-live videos, most of the engagement with Facebook Live videos comes after the live broadcast. Specifically, on average during the live broadcast, videos in their dataset receive 6.7 likes, 8.4 comments, and 0.54 shares; one day after broadcast, the engagement counts jump to 29.84 likes, 16.33 comments, and 1.33 shares (Raman et al, 2018). Lamenting that because as much as 41.5 per cent of all Facebook Live videos were never watched, the researchers suggest locally storing the video content on the broadcasters' mobile devices until viewers arrive to save network bandwidth and battery consumption. This recommendation, if taken up by Facebook Live, triggers a fundamentally different model of content circulation on the platform: one that resembles an on-demand service, where livestreaming videos without an audience are set free from the mobile devices that house them only if these livestreams fail to satisfy the conditions that make them 'live' in the first place. In other words, broadcasts are not broadcasts if they fail to cast upon a broad audience, and live videos are not live if their audience comes with a delay.

What is missing here? From a technical point of view, liveness seems to be synonymous with simultaneity: are there people watching at the other end, as the video is being recorded? Yet for liveness to come about, instantaneity also needs to be at play: a video trapped inside a mobile device simply cannot 'go live'. At the heart of what motivates the researchers of this study lies the unexamined intimate relationship between 'real-time' and sociality – be it to the event/performance, or to people – that colours the experience of liveness. The meaning of 'live' is always contrasted to and informed by the 'non-live'; it is because of this that the conditions under which liveness comes into being deserve disentangling. Probing into the apparent paradox of liveness on Facebook Live could tell us something important about our relationship with time and the technology that mediatizes that relationship. As we will see in the section that follows, liveness oscillates between instantaneity and simultaneity as it takes on multiple iterations contingent on platform affordances. Liveness as instantaneity transforms downtime as moments of disjuncture, and as simultaneity provides temporal structure for the tactical persistence of practices that are out of sync with the rhythms of institution and society.

Liveness and time: a tale of co-dependency

Liveness is a central category in media studies' concern with the question of time and media (Auslander et al, 2019). Early works on liveness in relation to performances and mediatization have recognized the liveness category as historically contingent: what is experienced or counts as 'live' on one medium at one point in time does not necessarily remain stable over time and across media (Auslander, 2012). The continued relevance of liveness as a technological feature (ontology), an experience (phenomenology), and a normative value (rhetoric) has prompted van Es (2017) to develop a method she termed 'constellation of liveness' – where liveness is conceptualized as a socio-technical construction whose multiple forms populate the changing media landscape as they become bound by the roles they fulfil in society. Following this approach, van Es (2017) suggests understanding liveness as oriented around newness: that liveness is indebted to the particular ways in which media are increasingly structured to demand attention from people now, rather than later. It is through the mechanism of liveness that media platforms proliferate in abundance: in an overcrowded media landscape, each medium is asserting its significance through an appeal to the live (Auslander et al, 2019).

But when and how is liveness demarked from the non-live? Van Es (2017) suggests that the domain of liveness is constitutive of metatext, space of participation, and user responses. Metatext refers to a collection of information about the platform itself as discursive sites, which could include platform features, promotional materials, or interviews with platform representatives. Space of participation is shaped by techno-cultural, economic, and legal forces. User responses, which comprise instances of reflection and commentary on the platform by users themselves, contribute to the meaning of liveness through the agency of users interpreting the liveness proposed by metatext. There is a multiplicity to liveness; it neither exists in a pure form nor comes in a range of degrees – liveness is contingent on a situational context as well as knowledge of what it is that is being made 'live'.

If liveness is multiple, so is time. Time with a capital T – clock-time, or universal time – is standardized in replicable units to provide a temporal structure to everyday life, but it is not the only way in which time is experienced. Nowotny (1989, 2019) describes *eigenzeit* – self-time – to capture qualitative changes in individual perception of time and the corresponding experience to the structuration society imposes on time. These changes are a result of acceleration – a phenomenon she conceptualizes not only as owing itself to science and technology, but also as contingent upon the cultural and social interconnections that are enabled, boosted, and expanded by technology. This acceleration also results in a more profound change: that in the relationship between lifetime and *eigenzeit*. Time seems to be out of joint for most of us: a 'deep-seated sense of unease and massive stress' is caused by the speed with which the world is hurtling forth – a speed that outstrips our biological, cognitive, neural, and mental capacities (Nowotny, 2019, p 70).

But technology also giveth what it taketh away. In revisiting *eigenzeit* almost 30 years after it was first conceptualized, Nowotny (2019) describes what she calls 'medial *eigenzeit*' as a technology-based set of options to satisfy the longing for the moment. Medial *eigenzeit* is accessible from everywhere with a mobile device – it is at once standardized and personalized, individually available, and yet socially connective. As she puts it:

> Immersing oneself in medial *eigenzeit* grants time to indulge in exchange with others. Rather than the conscious void that is being sought in the practice of mindfulness, time is full of information – about the world, about friends, even if these are 'friends' only in the social media sense; information about oneself and those parts of it that we want to share with others. It gives us a sense that we are incessantly engaged in communication with the entire world. (Nowotny, 2019, p 77)

In living with medial *eigenzeit*, downtime is in constant rehabilitation. Here, downtime as temporal voids is augmented with a constant anticipation for what comes next. The body engages with technology in ways that add layers to its inner temporality and modulate its experience of time. We actively work through boredom with our hands: scrolling through our Facebook feed, thumbing our frustrations on Twitter, double-tapping the images we like on Instagram, sliding our fingers across the screen to skip to the part of a video we want to watch, extending our index finger and thumb to zoom in, narrowing them to zoom out. Each of these haptic motions commands a different body temporality; they have been designed to compensate for the lack of tactile feedback inherent to flat-screen devices so that they can facilitate effective human–machine interface. Our tactual exploration of the external world relies primarily on the hand: the hand is voluntarily moved across a surface or manipulates an object so that it can obtain specific spatial and temporal information. Viewing these tactual explorations with technology in the context of downtime allows us to examine how embedded technological uses are in time: how time motivates these uses as it lends itself to transformation by these very socio-technical enactments.

Through these exploratory procedures, our haptic sense serves as an intermediary for our vision and audition (Jones, 2018). Haptic sensing is unique compared to other human senses in that it is bidirectional: as we reach out to discover the properties of the world, we perceive as much as we also act directly upon it. On occasion, we also reflexively act upon our own body. As I will discuss in the section that follows, the case of *diện chẩn* livestreaming practice entails both the hand actively working through boredom by engaging with technology (in the case of livestreaming audience) and the hand demonstrating its capacity to recuperate not only downtime, but also its own material body (in the case of both audience and livestreamers). I will focus on the 'constellation of liveness' in Facebook Live to demonstrate how, through the temporality of downtime, liveness is able to oscillate between simultaneity and instantaneity. The result of this oscillation is a reverberation of multiple enactments of liveness that are more than one, but not fragmented into many: even when simultaneity and instantaneity do not coincide, they echo in each other's aura in the facilitation of liveness. I will also, through my description of the case, unpack downtime both as an empirical phenomenon and as an analytical category to explicate the relationship between downtime and *eigenzeit* more broadly.

The case of *diện chẩn*: downtime, liveness, and the body

Diện chẩn is an emergent non-biomedical therapeutic practice. Non-biomedical practices, defined as therapeutic modalities that exist in separation but not isolation from biomedicine, remain widely popular throughout the world. Variably referenced in disparate literatures as 'traditional medicine', 'alternative medicine', 'complementary medicine', and 'unorthodox medicine' (see Chapter 3), these therapeutic practices continue to exist, expand, and evolve at the margin of scientific biomedicine. This marginal existence, however, is only partial; in practice, non-biomedical modalities actively adapt and incorporate scientific methods and sensibilities into their repertoire.

Non-biomedical modalities are not monolithic. There exist complex nested hierarchies of authority within these therapeutic practices. Non-biomedical modalities proliferate with a different temporality compared to scientific biomedicine; they ebb and flow through the totality of the highly structured, albeit pluralistic scientific enterprise. They rarely directly confront or challenge the logic of scientific knowledge; it is not in the interest of their survival to do so. As such, their temporality is also different from that of inaccurate understandings of scientific knowledge – the kind that would fuel conspiracy theories and eruptive events such as anti-vaccination movements. Inaccurate understandings of scientific knowledge and conspiracy theories are quick, short, reactive, and cyclical. The temporal currents of non-biomedical practices form new arms and channels as they branch out from the mainstream; new therapies and new interpretations of traditional texts are in constant negotiation with regulatory regimes, the traditions they build upon and veer off, and science with a capital S. What these new arms and channels lack in the authority that comes with established traditions, they make up for in their flexibility to adapt, hybridize, and reinvent themselves.

Diện chẩn is such an example. Behind this emergent Vietnamese non-biomedical practice, which has attracted an international following via the internet, is an obscure man named Bùi Quốc Châu, who claims to have single-handedly invented a new way to diagnose and treat most diseases through particular ways to massage the face. Particularly, different constellations of points on a human face, according to *diện chẩn*, are said to correspond to different organs in the human body. If these points are massaged correctly, the claim is that any and all diseases within the corresponding organs can be cured. For example, intense and frequent massaging of the mentolabial sulcus (area between the lower lip and the chin) using a *diện chẩn* tool is claimed to cure uterine fibroids, as the area is believed to correspond to the uterus in the female body. *Diện chẩn* claims to have gathered millions of followers in 35 different countries (Vu, 2020). My own documentation of this method shows that *diện chẩn* materials are available online in at least nine different languages (English, French, German, Italian, Polish, Portugese, Russian, Spanish, and Vietnamese). Bùi Quốc Châu's claim of originality and efficacy was once taken seriously by important politicians in the politburo in the 1980s. In 1988, Bùi Quốc Châu was sent to Havana, Cuba on a mission to both help promote 'Vietnamese medicine' to Vietnam's Communist ally in the Caribbean and to help him hone his craft through 'scientization' (Vietnam National Archive, 2020). The mission was not successful, however, and with the political turbulence within the politburo also came the downfall of *diện chẩn*: Bùi Quốc Châu's *diện chẩn* research centre in Ho Chi Minh city was later seized by the government, and Bùi Quốc Châu's subsequent attempts to gain regulatory recognition by the Vietnamese government proved futile. In 2003, *Lao Động* newspaper published an article alerting readers to the lack of scientific basis in *diện chẩn* as a method (VNExpress Online, 2003). In 2012, *Sài Gòn Giải Phóng* newspaper published a three-part investigation into *diện chẩn* and concluded that *diện chẩn* practice not only lacks scientific foundations, but that it could also be illegal (Sai Gon Giai Phong, 2012a, 2012b, 2012c).

In the sections that follow, I report on the results of my fieldwork in 2019 on *diện chẩn* practice in Vietnam and the US, where I observed and interviewed followers and practitioners of the method at their clinics and their homes, and over videotelephone applications. I also interviewed Bùi Quốc Châu himself, although his interview is not reported here. In so doing, I explore how downtime is drawn upon by interviewees to explain their engagement with the method, as well as the technologies that make the method readily and instantly accessible to them. I have given my interviewees pseudonyms to protect their identities. As *diện chẩn* moved away from the legal and scientific battles for recognition, it increasingly moves towards the internet, where its tactile propositions find resonance with the temporality of the mobile technologies on which it travels, as it intervenes the self-maintenance of the body and interrupts the temporalities of everyday life.

The main vignettes from my fieldwork are Thu, Lam, and Quang. Each of these vignettes illustrates distinct experiences of multiple liveness, medial self-time, and technology. Thu commits to a career in livestreaming *diện chẩn* therapy tutorials to transform downtime as a larger episode of personal crisis; yet the increasing intensity and scope of what she understands as appropriate for livestreaming is a transformation of downtime as disjuncture of the moment. Lam consumes these therapy livestreams to transform the downtime that comes with experiencing illness; his subsequent decision to pursue livestreaming as a producer both resolves the need to overcome downtime as residing between the action and inaction of everyday life and as an opportunity to translate a digital practice into urban mobility. Quang's experience with consuming therapy livestreams is similar to Lam's, yet his transnational mobility is tied to his need to recuperate time for a sick body that has been made to wait, away from home.

The *durée* of downtime

Thu is in her early 40s; when I met Thu at her apartment-cum-clinic in a brand-new apartment complex inside one of Ho Chi Minh City's latest urban development zones, the door was kept open. As I entered and introduced myself, Thu casually nodded her head to acknowledge my presence and asked me to wait in the clinic room. In the middle of the clinic was a long wooden table, surrounded by plastic chairs on all four sides. There was also a lone hospital bed pushed against the top right corner of the room, under a large window with a view facing the *Sài Gòn* river. As I sat down at the table on which dozens of tripods and smartphones were placed, I noticed that the clinic walls are filled to the brim with *diện chẩn* point chart posters that resemble acupuncture maps of pressure points on the body. I didn't mind the wait as there was a lot to take in; where point chart posters didn't fit, portraits of Bùi Quốc Châu and photos of him and his followers would enter to fill up what could otherwise have been some white space on these walls.

When Thu finally came in to begin our interview, I noticed that she had changed into her uniform – a light purple mandarin collared shirt with toggle buttons, which resembles traditional medicine doctor attire, and a large diện chẩn logo on her left chest. Two of her assistants quickly picked up the phones and tripods on the table to install a three-camera setup. I explained to her that it was her right as a participant to enjoy anonymity and to withdraw from the study at any point she so wishes. "It's OK, I don't want to be anonymous. I livestream everything I do here at this clinic every day. Someone will watch it, that's how I stay connected with my clients," said Thu.

And so our conversation began. Every time I came back to visit the clinic and talk to Thu's students and patients, our conversation would be livestreamed on Facebook. I later learned that this almost obsessive documentation and broadcasting of everyday events has become a ritual of sorts for all members of her 'crew'. Everyday events are livestreamed on Facebook precisely because they could be; the possibility of an audience is enough to justify the broadcast of an event, regardless of its perceived quality or intended purpose. And because Facebook automatically archives livestream recordings after the livestream has ended, Thu and her crew also see 'going live' as an important record-making activity. Thu has a university degree that allowed her to work for a few international companies for almost a decade, during which time she had the opportunity to practise her English and be exposed to foreign cultures, she assured me. Her radical turn to diện chẩn, a '100 per cent Vietnamese therapeutic method', coincided with major disruptions in her life: disillusionment with a 9 to 5 job that did not pay well, marital problems, the birth of her son, and a sudden but deeply felt need to reconnect with Vietnamese culture. She quit her job, moved back in with her parents, and waited for her life to turn around. As would be the case, Thu's mother happens to be one of Bùi Quốc Châu's original followers since the 1980s. Her mother, Ms Tuyet, would frequently travel South, leaving her and her father behind in Northern Vietnam during the 1980s and 1990s, to accompany Bùi Quốc Châu on various diện chẩn-related trips overseas. She said:

It was fate, when I felt the most stuck, unseen, and unfulfilled, my mother said maybe it was time I turned to diện chẩn. Not only can I take care of myself with this craft, I can even take care of thousands of other people all around the world. They watch me demonstrate, then they practise this [method] on themselves. They watch me practise it on other people, then they do the same on their families and friends. If it works, their families and friends would then practise it on themselves, then on their friends … it's an ever-expanding circle of care.

Thu's practice of *diện chẩn* has filled her downtime with activity on two different levels. During a significant episode of personal crisis – this is downtime on a lifetime scale – Thu turned to *diện chẩn* to pulsate the flatlining temporal rhythm in which she found herself. She said:

> This is a very dignified craft, before I became involved in *diện chẩn*, I would never dream of commanding a police officer or telling him to follow my instructions. A police officer! Can you believe it? One of my patients is a policeman. I told him to lie down on this bed and take off his shirt so I could perform *diện chẩn* on him to help with his cervical vertebrae. I livestreamed it on Facebook of course, you can always check it. People like him would never have given me the time of day in my previous life as a nobody. *Diện chẩn* has completely changed my life for the better.

Thu needed a sense of purpose; a purpose that can be achieved by doing something instantly, so as not to feel left behind. There is a certain indignity to being someone who waits in a culture of the instant. To sit around waiting is to be out of sync with modernity, with the habit of velocity that dictates how one should live their life; it is to be out of sync with time itself.

Downtime also comes with the experience of illness. Lam, who joined Thu's group from his hometown less than 200 km south of Ho Chi Minh City, was 19 years old when I met him. I sat down with him at a coffee shop near the clinic to talk about his introduction to *diện chẩn* on a separate occasion. As soon as the conversation began, Lam was comfortable enough to share that in his final year of high school, he discovered *diện chẩn* because he had haemorrhoids at the time and 'Western medicine' was of no help to him. Out of frustration, he looked up haemorrhoids cures on the internet and followed a few *diện chẩn* tutorials on YouTube, which according to him was able to help him manage the condition. He later discovered the growing number of *diện chẩn* communities on Facebook, Thu's included, and found out that he could take a *diện chẩn* class directly with Bùi Quốc Châu if he would make the trip to Ho Chi Minh City and pay the VND5 million (roughly USD220) tuition fee. When he finished high school, his score was not good enough for him to get into university; he figured that pursuing *diện chẩn* professionally – something he seemed to have a particular talent for – would set him apart from his high school friends, who were too busy "chasing grades and studying what they hated". With his parents' blessing, he moved to Ho Chi Minh City to embark on his journey as a *diện chẩn* professional. He said:

My main job in Ms. Thu's group is packing and sending *diện chẩn* tools to customers, as well as designing visual materials for social media. I won't lie, I was disappointed at first. I expected to be practising *diện chẩn* on patients right away, curing and helping people. After all, I took my classes with master Bùi Quốc Châu himself. But now I know that working these tasks gives me more confidence, more experience in communicating with people. Ms. Thu pays me well for someone with no diplomas to speak of. The people we help, especially people we met in a pagoda in *Bình Định* province on our *diện chẩn* mission trip, appreciate and respect us. I could not ask for a better job right out of high school.

If downtime for Lam is tied to both the experience of an illness that damaged his self-confidence and the anxieties of getting out of school without a clear direction, downtime for Quang, a Vietnamese-American in his mid-60s who had been living in California since 1973, is a matter of mortality. Having served in the South Vietnam army before Communist North Vietnam won the war in 1975, Quang had vouched to never return to Vietnam on ideological grounds. I met Quang and his family of four, together with two of his best friends in the US, at Thu's clinic on one hot December afternoon in 2019. He had decided to spend his winter break in Ho Chi Minh City studying *diện chẩn* with Bùi Quốc Châu and frequenting Thu's clinic to both 'hang out' and get Thu to help with his wife's chronic fatigue. Quang had been diagnosed with pancreatic cancer four months before this trip; a family relative in the US recommended that he looked up *diện chẩn* on Facebook and follow the livestreaming tutorials on there to help with his illness. "These people are legit, you know," Quang told me firmly:

I'm not one to be fooled. I know all this seems a little unconventional, but *diện chẩn* really works. I don't just uproot my family on a whim. My wife and I own a *phở* shop in Garden Grove, Orange County; it's not easy for us to leave the shop to our staff and come here for my treatment.

Quang and I had a long conversation, which was of course livestreamed on Facebook, as we watched Thu perform various *diện chẩn* massage procedures on his wife, Xuan, who is in her early 50s. In another room, An, one of Thu's assistants, was performing other procedures on Quang's friends, Toan and Lan, who are in their 70s and 40s respectively.

I had my doubts initially, as you can imagine. I live in the US, this kind of stuff is usually seen as quackery over there. I took the time to google 'dien chan' and 'scam' together. There was no result! But there were a lot of results for 'dien chan', in all kinds of languages, even Russian. All of these results sing praises about master Bùi Quốc Châu and Thu's group. That's how you know they are the real deal.

It was not my place to point out the flaws in his information appraisal strategy. Quang quickly became preoccupied with *diện chẩn*, practising it every day and closely following Thu's livestreaming videos on Facebook. He explains:

> The greatest thing about this method is that it allows you to be in charge of your own body, your own health. Western medicine takes away all that power from you. You go to the hospital and they let you die there. No dignity whatsoever. Obama made us pay premium prices for nothing. Trump is no better. Here you can practise on yourself, on your family, on your friends. Wherever it hurts, you control it with your own hands. There is true power in that ability.

The body cannot wait: the oscillation between instantaneity and simultaneity in liveness

If there is indignity in waiting around, there is enchantment in waiting for an object of desire: on the other side of waiting stands the promise of meaningful connections and the abolition of boredom. If waiting around is *eigenzeit* being out of sync with the times of others, waiting as enchantment ensures that recalibration is always an option. Liveness as simultaneity is the promise of this enchantment; as instantaneity, the promise of dignity: after all, to show respect is to not keep someone waiting. This double recalibration of liveness could act as an efficient time transformer as it enables social arrangements to veer towards the integration and assimilation of different temporal horizons and speeds. Making a sick body wait can be a painful and humiliating ordeal. A body recuperating itself from waiting by extending its primary tactual exploration part – the haptic hands – to touch, scroll, pinch, slide, press, massage, wave, gesticulate, is a body quite literally taking matters into its own hands. We cannot help sensing tactual sensibilities through our skin any more than we can help the passing of time; or as Bergson (2002, p 216) would put it: 'It is we who are passing when we say time passes.' Quang said:

> Thu is livestreaming all the time, so it's rare that I would run out of materials to learn. If not a tutorial then she'll be streaming her performance on someone, or introducing new tools that I can buy, or talking about *diện chẩn* in general. There is a significant time difference between Sai Gon and California, so sometimes I watch her livestreams

after the fact. Doesn't matter to me. She's very charming, Ms Thu. She has what it takes for this craft. She knows how to speak to people. Sometimes I watch the same video again and again; I would learn something new every time.

Xuan smiled at me as she sat up straight on the designated treatment bed so An could perform a range of massage techniques that were supposed to help Xuan with her chronic fatigue. She was never as involved as her husband Quang in the practice of *diện chẩn*, but remained supportive. "Quang is the kind of man who becomes obsessed really quickly. Whatever he chooses to pursue, he invests all his time and attention." "Was that how he pursued you?" giggled Thu, as she asked Xuan to move a little to the left.

Sure he did. But seriously, he is engrossed in this thing. Always on his phone watching videos, at the *phở* shop, at home, picking up the kids, before going to bed … One time I even asked if he's forgotten that he had a wife! He apologized by giving me these *diện chẩn* massages to help me with my back problem. It really did help. When he decided that we would come back to Vietnam so he could learn more about this method, I gave him my full support. We're all here, aren't we?

As downtime becomes recalibrated, it expands and transforms the structure of the everyday. Technology as an option with which to live through downtime has the capacity to weave downtime into the very fabric of time itself. As far as Thu and Lam are concerned, downtime has been permanently recalibrated; as long as they can livestream their works instantly, every day, they are producing digital materials that reiterate their newfound social prestige and rescue them from a previous kind of downtime: downtime as dwelling endlessly in a material world that turns against them, so that their bodies are not so much material facts, but manifestations of duration. 'It is we who are passing when we say time passes' (Bergson, 2002, p 216). Recalibrated downtime is a kind of medial *eigenzeit* that relieves the body from feeling its own weight. Without the technologies that transform, repurpose, and objectify time, we become time's vessel: the sick body feels this most emphatically. For Quang, every moment he otherwise would have spent worrying and feeling helpless is now an opportunity to engage both in a bodied practice that is already instantly available, and in a transnational community built on the mobilization of downtime. Quang's recalibrated downtime is living through medial *eigenzeit* that yearns for reconnection with the body in the moment and on its own terms. Quang told me when Thu and An were out of the room:

Look, I'm not delusional. I know there is no absolute cure to my cancer. But if there is something out there that helps, even just a little, of course I'd try. And so far, these exercises have really worked. I feel much better, bit by bit, every day. You know, me in front of my phone, in my palm, like this. She [Thu] presses (acupressure) point number 12 three times – I press point number 12 three times ... It's like I'm practising it with her. There is a kind of genius in that simplicity.

Liveness is not reducible to instantaneity, however. A recording of a live event is different from a non-live video recording, not only because it is experienced as such, but also because it requires specific temporal coordination from the livestreamer and the audience, as well as particular technological affordances to facilitate that liveness. Thu explained that as her audience base of *Việt Kiều* – a colloquial term referring to overseas Vietnamese – expands, she becomes more strategic about what kind of content to stream at which point of the day.

Most of these *Việt Kiều* live in California. That means our afternoon is their morning. I've realized that most of them are up and online at around 4pm our time. I try to schedule as many appointments with my clients in the afternoon around that time as possible, so they can wake up and see me in action. If that's not possible, I always prepare to give a live tutorial around their common problems, like back pain, migraine, heart diseases. Sexual problems are also common. Or problems with fertility. I listen to their problems and I show them a way to solve these problems. Their feedback is key to this process.

This feedback loop not only informs what should go live, it also informs the temporality of liveness. Encountering live videos is increasingly becoming a dominant feature in the Facebook experience: in 2017, one out of five videos on Facebook are live videos (99firms, 2023). The liveness of Facebook Live videos owes itself in large part to its platform logic: even though Facebook itself is not seen as a 'live' platform, its News Feed is commonly associated with liveness, both in popular discourse and by the platform itself (van Es, 2017). A Facebook Live video appearing on a user's News Feed therefore enjoys this double sense of liveness; the instantaneity of the event is relative to when the event becomes visible to the user. This crucial timing depends not on universal time, but on Facebook's News Feed algorithm – a techno-social artefact built on implicit and concealed implementations of network temporality. Facebook algorithms are proprietary and 'black-boxed'; while it is common knowledge that these algorithms are continually tweaked, a complete dissection of these algorithms is neither available nor possible. Some *metatext* about Facebook algorithms is available, however. Van Es (2017) reviewed the principles of temporal organizing of content on Facebook through two main algorithms, EdgeRank (for page post and status update personalization) and GraphRank (for application recommendation personalization, less relevant in our discussion). EdgeRank calculates an affinity score between Facebook users based on the number of interactions between the user initiating the connection (edge) and the viewing user, the weight of each edge type, and time decay – a measure that takes into consideration how long ago an edge was created. The newer the edge, the more relevant it is to the users involved: the higher the likelihood of the associated content to appear on News Feed. This elaboration of network sociality has an implicit built-in temporality, one that favours both instantaneity and simultaneity, although perhaps not of equal measures – there is no transparent way to tell. Given the dynamic nature of Facebook networks, due both to the constant modifications made to platform algorithms and to the trajectories of human relationships, organization of Facebook content is likely to oscillate between these two temporal qualities. The reverberation of simultaneity and instantaneity on all levels of this constellation of liveness – from platform temporalities to the multiscale downtime that carves out a *space of participation* where techno-cultural, economic, and extra-legal forces converge, and the everyday reflections and tactics of uses from users (or *user responses*) – circumscribe the domain of liveness on Facebook.

Downtime, recalibrated: enactments of liveness and their effects

Previous sections have shown that liveness is variously enacted rather than existing in a pure form that can readily be contrasted against the 'non-live'. These enactments oscillate between simultaneity and instantaneity: the decision to 'go live' on Facebook is made because it can be done instantly, just as the decision to watch a live recording is made because it is instantly available. Thu would livestream any and all activities happening in her clinic because her phones and tripods are at hand; Quang would watch all live recordings multiple times because they are made available to him instantly through his phone. Simultaneity becomes a character of second-order importance because it is thought to have been built into the platform affordances of Facebook Live. When there is a conscious attempt to coordinate simultaneity in Facebook livestreaming, the live event is demarked not from non-live events, but from other live events of a different temporality: it is an occasion in which simultaneity becomes of first-order importance. Thu's conscious shift in livestreaming strategy in response to her audience in California enriches her livestreaming practice with an added temporal layer, rather than restructures it so that it could align with real time. A live broadcast is made and watched precisely because it has been enacted as live, not because it corresponds with the temporalities of universal time via the technologies that remain faithful in ex-temporalizing time. Liveness does not happen in Time inasmuch as it happens in the enactments of itself – an enactment contingent on the moving pieces of liveness as a constellation. These varying experiences of 'live' not only help the body reconfigure its being-in-time as instantly and readily replenished with meaning and activity, but also fill these otherwise temporal voids – experiences of pure temporality – with shifting webs of temporal sociality.

Even though user enactments of liveness might contrast with the kind of liveness enacted by engineers and computer scientists (see again, Raman et al, 2018), liveness is not fragmented into many. Engineering livestreaming into Facebook – a platform whose temporalities already oscillate between simultaneity and instantaneity thanks to the algorithms that organize its content and condition its participation – is a task inevitably informed by this oscillation. There is a reverberation of this oscillation on three different levels: on the livestreaming feature itself, within the platform, and in the downtimes of its users. The result of this reverberation is a radical recalibration of downtime with technology: one in which the body as sensory central reaches out to its mobile technology to actively reconfigure its being-in-time. In the specific case examined here, the body also took a leap of faith to direct its haptic and tactile explorations onto itself – living with technology in a recalibrated downtime has allowed the body to recognize itself also as an entity to be acted upon, to be reworked and renovated.

While not all recalibration will entail this reworking of the body, the case examined here has outlined how this leap of faith is made possible not so much because of the newness or uniqueness of the practice *content* or the liveness *event*, but rather because of the *temporal reverberation* of downtime and liveness as enactments of the body and its technology. In other words, it is neither the uniqueness of *diện chẩn* as a method nor the novelty of livestreaming strangers massaging each other using odd-looking tools that allows the practice of *diện chẩn* to gain traction: the content and the event of liveness are expendable, owing themselves to the temporal reverberation in time, technology, and the body. This reverberation also carves out a temporal space for practices and enactments that are shunned by temporal structures of institutions and society to thrive: after all, downtime comes into being in the fractures between the mismatches of temporal regimes. Downtime and the insistence it puts on the body, which could mobilize both the production and consumption of livestreaming, are an often overlooked aspect of livestreaming practices. In the 'constellation of liveness' framework developed by van Es (2017), for example, liveness is a particular interaction between institutions, technologies, and people. It is through the analytical lens of downtime, as discussed in this chapter, that the mechanisms of how this interaction takes place can be traced. Enactments of liveness on Facebook are a result of temporal reverberations of downtime and liveness as enactments of the body and its technology, the result of which is a tactical temporal space that thrives at the margin of institutional temporal structures.

And yet there are inherent limits to this reverberation. The duration of liveness and downtime alike is limited, much like the finitude of lifetime. Recalibrating downtime in service of rescuing the present moment through engaging with liveness is but one of the many ways in which the body can reflect on its embedding in its lifetime – a reminder that clock time marches forward, unwavering. Quang recognized that his pancreatic cancer will eventually outrun his exercises, Thu recognized that she cannot out-generate tutorials for the growing conditions of her client base, and Lam recognized that at some point he will outgrow being the delivery boy for Thu's group. Any temporary unity between the self and its being-in-time at the behest of technology is intervened by its conflicted longing for the durability of human existence, which reminds the self of its ultimate precarity and eventual decay. Constant recalibration of downtime through enacting liveness is a tactical cheat that is able to seize little triumphs in between the cracks of temporal clashes, but is unable to keep any of them. The alternative temporal space created through the reverberation of downtime and liveness continues to thrive at the margin of more enduring temporal structures, even as it becomes front and centre in the everyday lives of those relying on it for survival.

A place for miracles: the internet as non-biomedical milieu

That *diện chẩn* practitioners and followers are able to continue practising this otherwise marginalized non-biomedical method via the creation of alternative techno-social spaces speaks to the nature of space as the product of interrelations and a sphere of contemporaneous plurality – as often experienced by internet users. The internet as a live middle space – a milieu of heterogenous eventualities willed into being together – is deeply embedded in a techno-social ecology which it helps shape and by which it is shaped. The productivity that arises from this milieu – in which people mobilize, cause others to mobilize, and make significant changes to their lives – is thanks to the increasingly seamless integration of digital technology into the rhythm of everyday life.

As non-biomedical knowledge continues to propagate and non-biomedical practices continue to evolve not through any single apparatus, but through an ensemble of multiple social media platforms, devices, temporal practices, and transnational networks, the internet emerges as a favourable milieu of development that can generate its own legitimacy. Within this milieu, any disruption to the rhythm of everyday life, even in the presence of illness, is voluntary and therefore manageable. Managing health and illness within this non-biomedical milieu means making oneself useful by posing the least amount of disruption necessary to domestic life through the means of voluntary self-surveillance and self-healing. This enables an ethic of good health as resting well within the agency of the individual, even as they actively seek out non-biomedical networks of support and care – which is articulated onto a system of learning and transfer of knowledge made available to the individual and their network through the medicalization of the moment. Existing outside of the temporal structure of institutions such as hospitals, rehabilitation centres, or laboratories, non-biomedical practices that translate well not only from historical and cultural ideas about health and illness from which they originate, but also into the temporal rhythm of the mundane every day, stand to persist as they continue to create and fill up spaces left unattended by the biomedical enterprise.

It is tempting to view digital traces (often understood as 'content') that, upon disembodied encounter through the opaque organization of platform algorithms, could be reduced to their informational properties – as either accurately or inaccurately informing the public about health and illness. This chapter and the following chapter argue that this reduction is unproductive as it ignores the deeply spatial ways with which people articulate their engagement with the internet as a techno-social system – as well as the spaces that the social processes behind these digital traces reflect and actively produce. An ecology-driven approach is better equipped to conceptualize the materiality and sociality attached to these digital traces. Understanding the internet as a non-biomedical milieu that embeds and conjoins physical as well as non-physical spaces crystallizes the temporal conditions it helps create – as well as the practices that thrive within these conditions.

In the next chapter, we will further explore how digital miracles are enacted in these spaces through the logic of play. In particular, we will turn to the charismatic Bùi Quốc Châu and his very elaborate – though misguided – articulations of digital technologies as miraculous media capable of carrying the mythical healing effects of the rituals he performs in front of his mobile phone screen, whose reflection is faithfully shown in his patients' screens across the sea. The world of technology as inscrutable systems, as such, enters the everyday world of human actors and re-emerges as magic: granting magical access to a previously closed world of sociality and accomplishing its magic by integrating people and things in a techno-supernatural sphere.

7

Curing as Play: The Internet as Miraculous Milieu

In the last chapter, we have seen how livestreaming technologies transform downtime and enable alternative temporal spaces, allowing social practices that are shunned by the temporal structures of institution and society to retune and continue to thrive at the margin of these structures and at the centre of the everyday. At the heart of this transformation is the collective experience of the internet as a space – as well as the playful nature of this experience. Spatial language infuses the way in which the internet is discussed in popular culture. From the famous adage 'On the internet, no one knows you're a dog' (Steiner, 1993), to allusions to 'cyberspace', 'online world', and 'global village', the internet is often understood as a place that is at once disembodied and yet spatially capable of bringing the world together (Graham, 2013). One goes 'on' the internet and 'to' a website in the English lexicon, as Graham (2013) points out, as if there is a singular virtual place equally accessible to all. Vernacular equivalents of the grammatical rules associated with the internet in the English language can also be found in Vietnamese – one goes 'up' or 'onto' the internet ('lên' mạng) or 'into' a website ('vào' web). As a space, the internet enables 'free flows of information' and is host to 'online communities'. These spatial elaborations of the internet often go unexamined as they structure, condition, and constrain conceptualizations and thus computer-mediated practices, as well as producing novel experiences of place.

While the internet as a space lacks apparent coherence and closure, it is nevertheless seen as stationary and mapped out from the user-infrastructure perspective: even though the internet is a little different every time we refresh our newsfeed, click on a link, or livestream a video, there is a finite set of tasks that users can execute and manipulate when they are online. As such, activities on the internet take on an ontic role; this ontic role informs the notion that internet problems require internet-specific solutions – a discourse easily misconstrued as separate from problems and solutions that are 'social', 'cultural', or 'political'.

This demarcation between technology and society is prominent in the framing of the mis/disinformation problem (Hwang, 2020). Although digital mis/disinformation hardly exists independently of the material technology that constitutes it, there appears to be a bifurcation of information as abstraction and technology as milieu. For example, the internet is often understood as a 'conduit' for health misinformation (Bode and Vraga, 2018); when this 'conduit' intersects with the 'health arena', experts warn of life-threatening consequences (Wang et al, 2019b). This intersection produces a kind of multiplicity that often combines already well-delineated territories; it therefore becomes intuitive to ask questions about the prevalence of misinformation on social media about a particular health-related issue (Chou et al, 2018), whether experts can mobilize their expertise in this new context (Vraga and Bode, 2017; Armstrong and Naylor, 2019), or indeed whether technology can mobilize itself to intervene in the new space it helped create (Ghenai and Mejova, 2018; Ma et al, 2016).

In this chapter, I explore *in vivo* conceptualizations of the internet as space – in particular, a miraculous space – by reporting on fieldwork conducted with the *diện chẩn* group over ten months between April 2019 and March 2020 in Vietnam and the US, where I observed and interviewed followers and practitioners of *diện chẩn* at their clinics and homes, over videotelephone applications, and through their activities on Facebook. It should be noted that there are a number of prominent conceptualizations of the internet that contend with a spatial conceptualization, such as the idea of a media ecology (Altheide, 1995; Fuller, 2007; Malpas, 2018), the arboreal model of a network with centres and peripheries (Wellman, 2001; van Dijk, 2020), or the rhizomic model of Deleuze and Guattari (Buchanan, 2007; Hess, 2008; Beck, 2016). The goal of this chapter is not to propose and defend an alternative position on the spatial qualities of the internet against these well-established models. Rather, it seeks to explain when and how the internet becomes a miraculous milieu – and how play as a *mode of mediated experience* contributes to the miraculous effects of livestreaming. The chapter also demonstrates that another kind of multiplicity – apart from the combinatory multiplicity of overlapping territories in health misinformation discourse – exists when we unsettle the implicit assumptions we make about space as stationary and mapped out, and instead see space as the product of interrelations, a sphere of contemporaneous plurality – as often experienced by internet users. Four vignettes have been selected below; they each represent spatial articulations that are most distinct from one another while being most representative of the articulations I've collected in my fieldwork.

Record-making as space-making: documenting miracles

We made acquaintance with Thu in Chapter 6 through her own account of downtime as a result of a significant episode of personal crisis – and as leader of a *diện chẩn* crew. In our first meeting at her clinic, I explained to her that it was her right as a research participant to enjoy anonymity and to withdraw from the study at any point she so wishes, only to be met with total indifference. She said:

> It's OK, I don't want to be anonymous. I livestream everything I do here at this clinic every day. Someone will watch it, that's how I stay connected with my clients ... This humble clinic you see here is nothing compared to the splendour of our following on the net (*trên mạng*), but I guess you already know that.

Every time I came back to visit the clinic and talk to Thu's students and patients, our conversation would be livestreamed on Facebook. These livestreams are automatically available as recordings for later viewing. I later learned that this almost obsessive documentation and broadcasting of everyday events has become a ritual of sorts for all members of her 'crew' – as well as other *diện chẩn* groups that I have been able to trace through Facebook and through my visits to BQC's own clinic. Thu explained to me that her compulsive livestreaming of *diện chẩn* activities is a form of record-making; it is as much a tactical undertaking as it is an act carried out precisely because Facebook has made the technology readily available:

> Why do I livestream my practice? I don't know, why not? I want to help people so the more people can watch what I do here the better. I help my patients get better every day, people should see it with their own eyes. As I practise the method on my patients, I also explain what I'm doing to the audience. They can watch and learn from what I do. This is like a bonus from my usual tutorial videos. Even if they cannot follow me when I treat my patients on video, they can look up the tutorial videos separately, using the keywords I mentioned in my demonstration livestreams. You know, you can re-watch all livestreams after the fact, and even search for them. A lot of people do. Sometimes it's a little difficult to find old livestreams, so we re-share it on our feed, or make new livestreams with slightly different storytelling. It's all really invaluable resource. The wisdom of Master Châu lives on in living videos like these.

This elaboration of livestreaming as record-making is attuned to the particular affordances of Facebook as a platform: far from being an ephemeral technology, Facebook Live videos are stored in perpetuity as a recording and can be revisited any time, much like pre-recorded videos. Affordances are the ways in which technologies enable and constrain potential behaviours, the conditions of which vary by perception, dexterity, and cultural and institutional legitimacy (Davis, 2020). They can be best understood as relational properties that mediate action possibilities. While technologies cannot force people into doing things, it is through the mechanisms and conditions of their affordances that actions are encouraged or discouraged (Bucher and Helmond, 2017; Ettlinger, 2018; Hanckel et al, 2019). What would have been private play – between Thu and her patients and students – became public broadcast not only for education, but also therapeutic entertainment.

While the act of going 'live' in this context might be spontaneous, the digital traces it leaves behind are perceived not as a platform by-product, but as premeditated footprints that can be, and will be, drawn upon as record. Record-making in this context is also space-grabbing. A record, once made, is 'stored' somewhere. While the metaphor of cloud computing – the imaginary that our data immaterially reside 'in the clouds' – has become ubiquitous in English-speaking contexts, the same does not apply in this context. It seems imperative that a techno-social site be constructed to augment the limited physical space that *diện chẩn* takes up: one that remains visible and accessible insofar as the act of record-making never ceases. Record-making is not automatic record-keeping, however. Some level of archival orientation is necessary for record-keeping to occur – in other words, for records to be systematically managed and distributed. While the need for record-keeping (maintaining and indexing resources) is frequently mentioned, its practice is hampered by the impulse to 'go live' (you can always make more videos), perceived audience expectation (people want a constant stream of new videos or they would lose interest), and platform affordances that discourage effective subsequent knowledge retrieval and organization (proprietary algorithms that prioritize livestream videos over other asynchronous broadcasts, achronological ordering of Facebook newsfeed). This trifecta conditions a dynamic sense of space-grabbing of the internet as constituted through interactions – of space as a product of interrelations constantly under construction. While record-keeping and, by extension, systematic knowledge management require a mastery and ordering of space as enclosure, excessive record-making is active, open-ended space-making. This active space-grabbing through the abduction of time – of creating spectacular events to compete for audience attention – is driven by a techno-social precarity that, while having an enabling effect, is just as daunting as existing precarities facing *diện chẩn*. Thu continued:

> Yes, I sometimes worry about the authorities. They have made it difficult for us in the past. News media are also very biased against us,

although recently they have softened their prejudice. The establishment sees us as unorthodox, as anti-establishment even. We're simply too avant-garde, even when Master Châu invented this method way back in 1980. But we are more ubiquitous than you might think. There are a lot of traditional medicine clinics who quietly practice *diện chẩn*. They don't advertise it publicly of course; they could lose their licences for that. Master Châu has long given up on the need to be recognized by the Agency of Traditional Medicine Administration. They are simply too old-fashioned. We do our own thing now, without the need for approval from anyone. The internet is wonderful like that. It leads us to the true path for *diện chẩn*: anyone can be free to practise *diện chẩn*, teach *diện chẩn*, interpret and appropriate *diện chẩn* for their own needs, all the while ignoring the noise from the naysayers.

As such, the internet is seen as a venue in which the multiple and simultaneous trajectories of *diện chẩn* would coexist in their full liveliness, regardless of underlying coherence. While the spaces for mainstream biomedical and non-biomedical practices alike are made and representational – qualities that cannot be detached from their history and context – the technosocial space for *diện chẩn* is that made of heterogenous impromptu acts of broadcast that are at once generative and elusive.

Sick and alone on the internet: the miracle of self-healing

We were acquainted with 19-year-old Lam in Chapter 6 as the errand boy for Thu's group, whose decision to move to Ho Chi Minh City to practise *diện chẩn* was inspired both by how the method helped him overcome his experience with haemorrhoids a few years prior – and subsequently, his conviction that he has a particular talent for curing diseases with the method. Lam explained to me in our first conversation what it felt like to carry the shame of illness as a teenager, and how he chose to manage the uncertainty of shame by losing himself to the internet:

> I couldn't talk to anyone about, you know, my haemorrhoids. I mean I eventually told my parents so they could take me to see a doctor, who was of little help … Since I was a kid I've always hated taking medications. It does no good to your body. I managed my condition by looking up cures on the internet, specifically using the keywords 'cures without medication' (*không dùng thuốc*). I found tons of such videos on YouTube, demonstrating how to cure my haemorrhoids by practising *diện chẩn* techniques. One video, two videos, then ten, twenty … I can't recall exactly how many videos I've watched and

practised along to. Must be a lot. There were days when I completely lost track of time; I would start practising to these videos after lunch only to stop for dinner. Then I would practise late into the evening before bed. I was hooked. You know what it's like to lose yourself to the internet, right? You get lost in there. Video led to video, then from YouTube I jumped to Facebook and Zalo (a popular Vietnamese messaging application). Just me and my phone, like this. Most of my friends waste their time on online video games, which is dumb. I learnt to cure myself and others from (từ) the net. It's a much more useful skill.

For Lam, the internet as a space might be characterized as providing the condition for therapeutic activities that generate time: time that can either be lost to wasteful online spaces or well spent being in spaces that help him with both his health condition and with finding a sense of purpose. The more time is spent on the internet, the larger the internet is envisioned as a space: to traverse and master a vast space, one needs to invest time. He maintained that his diện chẩn skills cured him of his haemorrhoids – the skills he later practised on his parents and extended family to help them with all their health problems to convince them of his unconventional career choice – and that the internet gave him an alternative space to explore where his abilities might best be invested. While Lam's individual experience of illness might have seemed isolated and isolating – that of an embarrassed young man practising along to obscure YouTube videos alone in his room – there is a great deal of sociability in Lam's experience of health subjectivity. This sociability is attributable to the spatiality with which the internet is thought of: Lam hardly noticed how time was passing as he immersed in a space of multiplicity – of the mobile technology he held in his palm, of the platforms he savvily navigated, of the connections he made through these platforms which eventually materialized into his mobility into the city. Lam's subjective experience with his health conditions was, therefore, not an internalized succession of sensations where the different points on his face were correctly massaged to somehow produce the effect of curing his haemorrhoids – an experience of pure temporality – but that of a relational nature, and his experience is therefore also spatial.

The heterotopic internet and the miracle of reconciliation

We made acquaintance with Quang in Chapter 6 as a returning Việt Kiều (overseas Vietnamese) dealing with prostate cancer, whose return to Vietnam was particularly meaningful as it was his first since his decision to live in exile. Quang and I had a long conversation as we watched Thu perform various diện chẩn massage procedures on his wife, Xuan, who is in her early

50s. In another room, An, one of Thu's assistants, was performing other procedures on Quang's friends, Toan and Lan, who are in their 70s and 40s respectively. Quang quickly became preoccupied with *diện chẩn*, practising it every day and closely following Thu's livestreaming videos on Facebook in a fashion similar to how Lam found himself 'lost' in a space of his own making. When he felt that the progression of his conditions required an intervention more radical than practising to Thu's paid online tutorials, he decided to make the trip to Vietnam for the first time in 46 years.

I'm not exaggerating when I say it's *diện chẩn*, Master Châu, and Ms Thu here that got me to go back to Vietnam. I no longer have any family here ... I might as well be a stranger in a strange land. The community I found in *diện chẩn* reminds me of a Vietnameseness that is rooted in traditional wisdom. Traditions, as you know, are free of politics. When you innovate a tradition, such as a medical tradition, you bring Vietnameseness to the world. Traditions have to be innovated where they started, so to speak. And then brought overseas. You cannot have real Vietnamese traditions in the US, for example. We're Vietnamese over there, but we also had to be Americans. It's a different kind of community. Once I'm in Master Châu's advanced *diện chẩn* class, I found a community almost immediately. People practised the techniques on me, and let me practise on them. It's easy when the culture is already there and you just become part of it. My treatment with *diện chẩn* is even more effective when I'm here.

The internet as a space of emplacement – of rhizomic assemblages, circulations of knowledges, including subjugated knowledges, and of transnational relations – also has the capacity to facilitate physical mobility and offer alternative possibilities in the production of space, though not seamlessly (Chung et al, 2018). Quang's decision to travel to Vietnam as a physical, territorial extension of the online space which augmented his everyday life in the US is one made on an understanding of space as absolute locations, as things in their places, and for Quang the place for *diện chẩn* is Vietnam. The internet, in this context at least, is what Foucault called a heterotopic space (Foucault, 1966, 1984) – a conceptualization of space that Foucault proposed through brief thumb-nail sketches and examples rather than resolving in a coherent way (Johnson, 2021). Foucault (1984, p 3) describes heterotopias as counter places, as an 'effectively enacted utopia in which the real sites, all the other sites that can be found in a culture, are simultaneously represented, contested and inverted'. Foucault uses the example of viewing his own reflection in a mirror. From one perspective, Foucault's reflection is in a placeless place, a utopia that exists in an 'unreal' place. But from another perspective, it is also a heterotopia: a mirrored image that does exist as a counteraction to Foucault's own position, where he is reconstituted in another place that is connected to the space around it. Cyberspace and platforms such as Facebook have been explored as heterotopias by various authors (see Rymarczuk and Derksen, 2014). Foucault's heteretopia for *diện chẩn* evokes a picture of juxtaposing spaces and sites that are 'other' to one another (Vietnam, America, the *diện chẩn* clinic), brought together through the internet and placed in the same 'garden', to use one of Foucault's examples, although they are in themselves incompatible. On this heterotopic internet, people and ideas that are otherwise unconnected connect; individual habitus, however, plays an important role in enabling these connections. In drawing on spatialized notions of 'home' and 'tradition', Quang is able to navigate and negotiate his personal health crisis away from the sight of his 'host country'. Vietnam, as such, is constructed anew as a bundle of ties that can be assembled and reassembled, rather than as a static storage space of Quang's personal memories. The internet as a heterotopic space is neither a coherent zone of consolation nor a chaotic sphere where 'anything goes'. It acts more appropriately as a mirror in the Foucauldian sense (Foucault, 1966, 1984); rather than being a reflective surface which closes representations of the social system in which it is a part, the internet discloses one's own social habitus and in so doing destabilizes senses of national territory as made and unchanging. Its disruptive impact on the way in which Quang confronts and manages his illness lies not in the way it seemingly mixes the profound with the profane – hence the framing of a 'battleground' for truth against misinformation – but in how it creates situations where Quang was forced to choose between a series of incompatible positions. As the internet recedes from its position in the foreground as an interface and into the background of everyday life, it flattens out the space of the techno-social and smoothens experiences of displacement: Quang quickly established a sense of community in Vietnam even as he found himself "a stranger in a strange land". Quang was adamant that his *diện chẩn* skills were upgraded thanks to his being in Vietnam, which subsequently helped with his condition. Perhaps similar to Lam, Quang's experience came less as a result of pure temporality – of therapeutic techniques perfected and generating a felt impact on Quang's body – and more as a spatial experience of being in the relational and dynamic techno-social spaces of his own making.

The miracle man himself: the internet as a conduit of healing power

Shortly after my first visit to Thu's clinic, she offered to introduce me to Bùi Quốc Châu at his residence. We sat down in his office on the second floor of his villa, tucked away in a small alleyway in Ho Chi Minh City. On the ground floor, people were sitting in the foyer waiting to see Cuong, one of Bùi Quốc Châu's sons, who is the practitioner on call for the day. The furniture would be moved around at night, Thu explained to me, so Bùi Quốc Châu could teach advanced *diện chẩn* classes in the same room where Cuong was diligently massaging his patients using strange looking tools that can be bought in an adjacent room. Bùi Quốc Châu is remarkably lively for a man in his late 70s; he would, however, get quite grumpy when I would occasionally try to steer him back from his incessant reminiscence of the past. Bùi Quốc Châu has many wild stories to tell; where his stories lack in clarity, they make up for in intricate details, punctuated with random mentions of French philosophers and famous Vietnamese politicians. As we talked about his overseas following – which is largest in Italy and Spain – and how technology helped him stay connected with them, he assured me that digital technologies do more than just help him popularize his invention:

I recently cured a whole family in Germany of back pain. Father, mother, and their son. You heard me, they're in Germany. Yes they are Vietnamese-Germans, the *Việt Kiều*, but I cured them while they are in Germany, not while they are visiting here. You ask me how? It's through this phone right here. They were practising my tutorials for back pain for weeks without any results, so they called me up using Zalo to ask for help. I asked the mum to show me the son's back on video. I then cured him through the videocall using my psychic energy through my palm. Just like I would if he was here physically. The phone carries my energy, you know. It travels through the internet, to Germany. You know, 4G technology these days, it's quite marvellous. He got better instantly. Only I can perform such a miraculous feat.

Following his early unsuccessful endeavours in legitimizing *diện chẩn* through scientization, Bùi Quốc Châu's turn to the supernatural and spirituality through claims and stories that would grant him quasi-sainthood status appears to have coincided with his core group's adoption of new technologies. While he does not manage his own social media presence, Bùi Quốc Châu regularly uses his smartphone to make direct contact with his overseas following, as well as taking photos and videos of *diện chẩn* events for his own record. The internet as a space accessed through the portal that is his mobile device is understood as one that is suitable for conveying therapeutic energy, which allows him to include internet-based activities into the rhythm of his everyday practice. In this transcendent interpretation of digital technologies as part of an ecosystem that allows invisible forces to make a direct impact on the human body from afar, the internet becomes a domesticated space: a space invented by science, but shaped in ways that accommodate the goals and desires of people engaging with that space. The internet is also understood as possessing special qualities that can facilitate the therapeutic experience; while these qualities might not be intrinsic to the technological infrastructure per se (not everyone can perform these 'miraculous acts'), they can nevertheless be activated through the performance of certain rituals in particular events. The choice to activate these special qualities is both utilitarian (the situation demands such a performance) and marked by deeply held beliefs about the relational nature of well-being, as well as the purpose and power behind new technologies. When the internet is successfully mobilized as such, it is further 'blackboxed' – the more effectively the internet is constructed as a conduit for healing energies, the more opaque and obscure it becomes, thus giving way to supernatural interpretations of the internet as embedded in existing webs of signification. The internet, once imagined as a non-physical space, lends itself to associations with the spiritual, immaterial world that has been purged from the biomedical gaze upon the body, yet ever present in the way in which the body experiences the world of which it is a part.

Discussion

This chapter has documented the ways in which in vivo spatial imaginations about the internet turn it into a favourable milieu for medical practices outside of the biomedical institution to persist. Here, themes of religio-morality and transnational material sociality resurface as indexes of space: as a conduit capable of carrying healing power and as a heterotopic space of emplacement. Bùi Quốc Châu is adamant about the capacity of the internet carrying the mythical healing effects of the rituals he performs in front of his mobile phone screen, whose reflection is faithfully shown in his patients' screens across the sea. Perhaps this sort of thinking is better articulated as the dialectic between technology and magic: the magical feats of the transformation of the arrangement of everyday life and the bewitchment of exercising authority through and over technology bring about a sense of gratification that cannot be otherwise described. The world of technology as interface and inscrutable systems as such enters the everyday world of human actors and performs in magical ways: granting magical access to a previously closed world of sociality and accomplishing its magic by integrating people and things in a techno-supernatural sphere. What is visible through technology only makes what it renders invisible even more magical: the immediacy of connection, the freedom and control our phones afford through tactical manipulation that translates into social and bodily effects – *creatio ex nihilo*, the techno-supernatural solution to a very worldly yet otherwise indomitable problem: that of mortality. Bùi

Quốc Châu's magical claims of curing patients via technology, where he sees the internet as a medium that allows him to employ quasi-physical magical powers to intervene (causally) on the conditions of his patients who live overseas, is perhaps more symbolic than he makes it out to be: phone screens cannot transfer or emit physical force from one human body to the next. Anthropologist Alfred Gell takes the view that magic as an adjunct to technical procedures persists because it serves 'symbolic' (or cognitive) ends (Gell, 1988). He connects the domain of magic-making with play: to him, magic, which sets an ideal standard, is not to be approached in reality, yet towards which practical technical action can be oriented. When children play, they provide a continuous stream of commentary on their own behaviour (for example, now I am doing this, now I am doing that, and now this will happen ...). Gell likens this to the format of spells, where reality is constantly idealized; the unrealizable reality of a child likening themselves to an airplane (with arms extended, and the appropriate sound effects and swooping movements), he argues, is both never confused with actual reality and at the same time sets the ultimate goal towards which play can be oriented, and in the light of which it can be intelligible and meaningful. Bùi Quốc Châu forcing his 'internal energy' out through his palms over his phone screen while narrating the impact of his actions can perhaps be likened to a child transforming themselves into an airplane in Gell's example.

In the spatial experience of Quang with the internet, the internet discloses his own social habitus and in so doing destabilizes senses of national territory as made and unchanging. As the internet recedes from its position in the foreground as an interface and into the background of everyday life, it flattens out the space of the techno-social and smoothens experiences of displacement: Quang quickly established a sense of community in Vietnam even as he found himself "a stranger in a strange land". Quang's dormant network ties, once reactivated, facilitate transnational mobility, and recover the effects of relational decay as a result of his exile. Far from only being reactivated when needed, the ties with Vietnam that Quang re-established through his engagement with *diện chẩn* fostered a renewed sense of belonging as well as an experience of reconciliation. The timing of this reactivation is crucial for this effect to have taken place: in living with a terminal disease under conditions perceived as hostile against his recovery in the US, the weak dormant tie that Quang has with Vietnam becomes a strong active tie that helps him and his family navigate this complicated experience. Transformative experiences of the kind that Quang went through here (uprooting his family, returning to Vietnam for the first time in 40 years, committing to the practice of *diện chẩn*) are perhaps likely to happen with such an extreme life event (being diagnosed with advanced pancreatic cancer). However, social media directly enabled this experience by providing explicit reminders to reconnect with dormant ties (Vietnamese-language content is more accessible to first-generation Vietnamese Americans like Quang, whose command of English does not meet his needs in the current situation) and create renewed awareness of their existence (through the emergent, tactical livestreaming practice of *diện chẩn* on Facebook). The social lives of digital miracles, as such, temporalize and spatialize in and through the technologies that mediatize them.

Epilogue: Curing at the Digital Edge

To the extent that internet cures are not online health misinformation, they resist the logic of intervention as problem-solving precisely because they provide resolution to problems that otherwise remain indeterminate: digital inscription of miracle cures as record-making and record-keeping, transnational networked sociality that emerges out of the increasingly datafied environment of executable text, the reconfiguration of downtime into connectedness and belonging, and the creation of an alternative miraculous space for therapy as a playful activity. The crowdsourcing of miracle cures happened organically via social media as an intermediary for matching community needs with community capacity; that the longevity of these online groups enables *post hoc* creation of datasets that can be explored computationally, that the dynamic knowledge-making processes that unfold on these groups become fully open to view thanks to platform affordances – are secondary to the pre-digital social dynamics that drove these practices forward. These secondary utilities, however, came to solidify and legitimize these practices in an ecology of datafied behaviour; in this process, these utilities also transformed the expectation around what it means to engage with miracle cures. If seeking herbal cures for cancer, for example, used to mean coming to a *lương y* ('doctor of good conscience') for advice, or to a herbal store to purchase *thuốc gia truyền* recipes ('family transmission' recipes) and coming away with instructions that are based on socially sanctioned expertise, increasingly people are taking to social media to work out the details of these bodies of knowledge both in response to emergent health concerns and to enact the work of care. That it became acceptable and even desirable to carry out this kind of work in such a digital context is a by-product of the historical continuation of practices that never quite ceased to exist in the first place – and also of emerging forms of sociality as compositions of meaning via digital platform affordances.

Miracle cures proliferate at the digital edge in ways that are very important to their survival: in languages that skirt the technical capabilities and political will of regimes of automated platform content moderation, as esoteric discourse that defies easy categorization, in formats that are prioritized for the imperative of platform profit, and at a temporality constantly recalibrated to accommodate self-time/*eigenzeit*. The digital edge, as such, is a threshold space – one that connects and distinguishes different digital activities while functioning as a source of movement for their mutual transformations. The palliative function of the internet in relation to digital miracles operates not in the accuracy, the speed, or the variety of its information – but rather in the way it creates thresholds for the transformation of miracle practices as personal, but also societal and technical, endeavours. From digital inscription of cures to public deliberation of how these cures fit into modern scientific classifications of ailment, from live broadcasts of miracle cures to delayed visits and revisits of livestreamed videos, from the miraculous effects of enacting miracle cures over distance with technology to the admission that perhaps miracles lie in the overcoming of distances to go back home as a family – the internet acts as a facilitator of miracles not as divine interventions, but as transformations to existing social practices. These transformative effects are compelling because they actualize imagined possibilities that otherwise would lay dormant in pre-digital enactments of miracle cures: that inscriptions of knowledge could be quickly and cheaply reproduced with fidelity at scale, that communities in exile could draw on familiar resources and support from the homeland, that the loneliness and indignity of falling ill could be overcome with an enchanted object one keeps on one's body, and that practices that are shunned by the more lasting institutional temporal rhythms could one day find an avenue for their renewed popularity.

To the extent that my insistence on an agnostic treatment of the truth claims behind the miracle cures presented in this book can be read as a critique of the mis/disinformation paradigm, it is a critique not against the usefulness of the paradigm per se, but rather against its porous and often unarticulated conceptual boundaries. The strategic essentialization of mis/disinformation in contemporary social research has allowed social scientists and humanities researchers to form alliances with their colleagues in the technical sciences to work towards the common goal of bringing order to an information environment muddled with aberrations. This characterization of our collective information environment is useful for the framing of a number of emergent issues, such as computational propaganda that weakens informed decision-making in liberal democracies, rumours and gossips about individuals that cause harm on their reputations and well-being, inaccurate information about vaccine efficacy that compromises public health initiatives, and so on. The formulation of refutable claims, followed by demonstrable harms and feasible interventions, is at the heart of how the mis/disinformation paradigm operates. Miracle cures, on the other hand, persist at the digital edge – as edge cases that cannot be adequately explained away by the dominant mis/disinformation paradigm and always at the cutting edge of new platform affordances, edging out new spaces at the margin of digital platforms. On the digital edge live people who not only find the conditions of the edge hospitable and therapeutic, but also seize this space of opportunity to continually reinvent their miracle practices. In recognizing the persistent existence of miracle cures at the margins of digital platforms, we are prompted to critically engage not only with the limits of disciplinary frameworks around information – but also the futility of attempting to eliminate or regulate these practices, given their resilience and cultural significance throughout history. If we were to ever grapple with the complexity of our information environment – a sentiment often invoked to justify concerted interventions on information disorders – we need to consider the edges, the miraculous, and the non-biomedical for what they are and not what we seek to marshal them into being.

APPENDIX 1

Topic Modelling Result Summary

Table A.1: Topics generated and their top 20 terms

Topic	Share % M (SD)	Top 20 terms (translated)
Topic 1: TM in context of formal national health care	3.33 (0.67)	Limited time, Curcumin, Seniority, Ranking, Two-week period, Bcl-2 protein family, Tràng phục linh (Colitis medication), Namo amitabud, Bảo an khang (Name of insurance scheme), Cutleaf groundcherry, Sickness, Tiger bone glue, Gathering, Half portion, Short course, Corn, Dental care, Russia, Kidney stone, Geoduck
Topic 2: General principles of TM	3.84 (1.02)	Local dialect, Quality, Ease, Human organs, Equilibrium, Blood veins, Medical effects, Fruits, Human anatomy, Egg, Cashew, Selection, Alternative, Kidney, Vinegar, Good quality, Pepper, Immersion, Softness, Food dish
Topic 3: Knowledge sharing as advertising for direct sales	2.67 (0.57)	Symptom, Dragon's tongue leaf, Phlegm, Service, Human back, Tuber fleeceflower, Southern medicine, Tomorrow, Once a day, Circumstances, Plant processing, Plant scouting, Inbox, Knowledge, Medicine, Parasite, Recipe, Soda, Lymphatic system, Frequency
Topic 4: TM as religious philanthropy	3.31 (0.18)	Seafood, Frequency, Healing, Buddhist monk, Fruit, Phlegm, Basic, Consequences, Philippines, Yao people, Species, Hua Tuo, [Redacted username], Favour, Variety, Tree trunk, Plucking, [Redacted username], Sharpness
Topic 5: General childcare advice	2.21 (0.46)	Blanket, Hotness, False daisy, Homegrown, Fibraurea leaf, Table, Standard, Correction, Determination, Ground substance, Average, Seeing, Thread, Malignant hyperthermia, Chickenpox, Addiction, Childhood, Vân Hồ (a district in Sơn La, Vietnam), [Redacted username], Faeces
Topic 6: TM as lifestyle	4.39 (1.04)	Blowing, Multitude, Avoidance, Shower, Tickling, Discovery, Leanness, Gypsum, Moisture, Sleep, Territory, Udumbarra flower, Backside, [Redacted usersame], [Redacted username], Atherosclerosis*, Vinegar*, Prevention, Fine meal, Miracle

Table A.1: Topics generated and their top 20 terms (continued)

Topic	Share % M (SD)	Top 20 terms (translated)
Topic 7: Dietary benefits of traditional plants and call for direct sales	4.26 (1.42)	Sabah snake grass, Digestion problems, [Redacted username], Contrast, Ray, Year, Condensed, Tonsillitis, Pneumonia, Instructions, [Redacted username], Tomorrow, Soup, Red blood cell, Effectiveness, Zalo (a Vietnamese messaging application), This, Body, Gift, [Redacted username]
Topic 8: TM as dietary supplements	3.21 (0.44)	Vietnamese ginseng, Brand name, An Tôn (a former village in Vĩnh Phúc district, Thanh Hoá province), Alleviation, Negativity, Hihi, Vitamin B12, Body temperature, Sympathy, Small dots, Familiarity, Chinese mesona, Falling, Western, Fairy, Cashew, Cornea, Half portion, Intermediate, Men
Topic 9: TM as narratives	4.02 (1.32)	Medicality, Hour of the pig, Desire, 30 minutes, Publishing request, Once upon a time, Brothers and sisters, Death, Heat, Stop, Flanovoid*, Pencil cactus, Steaming, Cannabis, Seeds, Paper-thin, Medicine, Ingredients, Country, The Americas
Topic 10: TM in family health	3.75 (1.02)	Rice wine, Lightness, Eternity, Itchiness, [Redacted username], [Redacted username], Bastard children, Tropics, Warmth, Calmness, Sand, Cashew, Sweetness, Computer, Beauty, Menstrual cramps, Tumour, Household equipments, Substance
Topic 11: Ethnic variations in TM	1.09 (0.43)	Peeling, Gold apple, Career, Cardboard, Socks, Body part, Support, Satisfaction, Lâm Thao (a Northern province in Vietnam, also name of a fertiliser brand), [Redacted username], Solasodine*, Peony, Thuốc Nam Phong (rheumatism medication), Promotion, Noel*, Infection, Doctor Triệu Thị Thanh (a Yao doctor), Clots*, Magnesium, Zinc
Topic 12: Managing alcohol addiction	2.14 (0.98)	Wood, [Redacted username], Body, Sickness, Pearl, Retrogade ejaculation, Baldness, Darkness, Trick, Movement, Bad luck, Thuỷ Ngàn (alcohol addiction medication), Bad temper, Vitamin K, Confession, Infection, Folliculitis, Craziness, Below*, Hemorrhoids
Topic 13: Shaming uses of TM	1.30 (0.40)	Beta-Sitosterol*, Shrimp paste, Speed, Pomade, Technology, Space*, Sterculiaceae*, 6 years, Monoglucoside*, Rarity, Precipitation, Suppression, News, Mood, Bookstore, Country bumpkin, Reasoning, Morning sickness, Occasionality, Belief
Topic 14: Managing mental health among overseas Vietnamese	2.23 (0.34)	America, Wormwood, Rowatinex*, Hatred, Juice, Contact, Heaviness, Thankfulness, Isothiocyanate, Insomnia, Anxiety, Kohlrabi, Rhythm, Sunglasses, Translation*, Participation, Bruises, Borrowing, Vacuum, Sickness

(continued)

Table A.1: Topics generated and their top 20 terms (continued)

Topic	Share % M (SD)	Top 20 terms (translated)
Topic 15: Managing smoking addiction with TM	2.36 (0.26)	Antonin Seipin★ (supposedly Russian doctor), Sleep, Vontaren★, [Redacted username], Gấc seeds, Bird, Walking, Dog blood, Hunger, 70 years old, Rheumatism, Water, Spine, Chicken, Picture, Gift, Food, Thankfulness, Heaviness, Intern
Topic 16: Cardiovascular health and overseas Vietnamese	2.26 (0.42)	Dick★, [Redacted username], Kkkkkkk, Untimely diagnosis, Shred, Penis, Garden, Combination, Announcement, Contradiction, Urging, Vitality, Hole, Hematology, Acceleration, Withdrawal, Visa★, Blood veins, Good reputation, Cikan (heart health supplement)
Topic 17: Anti-infective plants and pain management	2.00 (0.48)	La Gi (small town in Bình Thuận, Southern Central Vietnam), Common Purslane, Admin, Surplus, Usefulness, Salonpas, Indigenousness, Natural antibiotics, Summer, Autumn, Aches, Flower, Catching wind, Exercise, Trần Hưng Đạo (name of a street), Mink★, Bloodline, 100k, Boil
Topic 18: Cautionary tale against misuse of TM	1.57 (1.07)	Body, Women, Buying, Asking, Extra, Wine, Strength, Usage, Cancer, Diagnosis, Death, Sugar, Men, Friend, Steambath, Weekly, Turmeric, Tea, Derris
Topic 19: Men's sexual & reproductive health	3.42 (1.44)	[Redacted username], Dry-zone mahogany bark, Expenses, Cure, Scabies, Effectiveness, [Redacted username], Researcher, Materials, Archipelago, Regret, Prevention, Amber, Gossypol★, Indian goosegrass, Testicles, Limonene★, Hygiene, Schefflera heptaphylla, Pedology
Topic 20: Food as medicine	3.84 (0.24)	Food with 'cold' properties, Fermented tofu, Money, Duck meat, Area, Cash flow, Contradiction, Sickness, Interaction, Diaper, Method, Water, Bear gallbladers, Springing, Medical practice, Pig, Mother, Reference, Honey, Hybridity
Topic 21: Agrarian lifestyle as healthy lifestyle	2.28 (0.28)	Mushroom, PDR★ (Physician's Desk Reference), Happiness, Moment, [Redacted username], Tongue, 50 years, Buffalo, Quảng Ninh (a Northern province in Vietnam), Boil, Salt, Flies, Fullness, Applying ground leaves over wound, Shampoo, Class of plants, Fruit tree, Tea, Eating habits, Từ Sơn (a village in Bắc Ninh, a Northern province)
Topic 22: Buddhist lifestyle as healthy lifestyle	1.94 (0.12)	Suffocation, Digestion, Vegetarianism, Piper lolot leaf, Proof, Cần Thơ (a province in Southern Vietnam), Namo amitabud, Tree stump, Black bean, Studying overseas, Brain, Today, [Redacted username], The truth, Boat★, Taking medication, Storytelling, Adrenal gland, Happiness and Prosperity, Body organ

Table A.1: Topics generated and their top 20 terms (continued)

Topic	Share % M (SD)	Top 20 terms (translated)
Topic 23: Discussions on the origins and originality of Vietnamese medicine	3.14 (1.73)	[Redacted username], [Redacted username], Patent, Clutching, Usage, Southern territories, [Redacted username], Better quality, Ethnic minorities, Lips, Determination, Admin approval, Destiny, Tuệ Tĩnh Đường Liên Hoa (a TM dojo in Huế, Central Vietnam), Trịnh Hoài Đức (18th-century historical figure), [Redacted username], Coach bus, Malt, Pounding
Topic 24: Processes of preparing plants as medicine	1.62 (0.29)	House yard, Đống Đa (a district in Hà Nội), 6 months, Chromatophore, Purity, Daytime, Itchiness, Sleep, Nutrition, Rice wine, Oxygen, Chaff-flower, Gastrict acid, Bowl, Citizen, Fermenting and Drying, Purpose, Afternoon, Ribs, [Redacted username]
Topic 25: Emergency childcare advice	1.37 (0.43)	Tools and equipments, Baby colic, Examination, Squeezing, Amount, Inner body, Selection, Sharp pain, Binystar (baby colic medication), Liking, Roseola, Couch, Lung, Dollar, [Redacted username], [Redacted username], Alkaloid*, Statistics, Ceylon hill gooseberry, Mothers
Topic 26: Negotiating sales of medicinal plants	2.35 (0.44)	Hedyotis*, Willow bark, [Redacted username], Parasite, Personal taste, Family recipe, Blue, Middle, White, Negativity, Experience, Lingao County, Savings, Colitis, Eel, Storm, Feet, Virginity, Post office, Quality
Topic 27: Negotiating shipping methods and sales of medicinal plants	2.13 (0.72)	[Redacted username], Shade trees, Bank, 350k, Carboxymethyl cellulose, Peanut, Miracle, Flagellate, Hà Nội, Incomprehensibility, Index finger, Stemona tuberosa, Concurrence, Long Biên (a district in Hà Nội), Dear friend, Billards, Hoàng Công (coach bus brand), Square, Birds, Wrapping cloth
Topic 28: Gastroenterology health	2.62 (0.51)	Recipe, Sugar beets, Investment, [Redacted username], Business, Gastralgia, Eating*, Falling off, Country, Family recipe, Discussion, Flatulence, Macau, [Redacted username], Urination, Guava, Stinkvine, Effect, [Redacted username], Money
Topic 29: Mental health and longevity	2.00 (0.62)	Reason, 100-year-old, [Redacted username], Greetings, Finickiness, Reasoning, Well-wishing, Anolyte, Acute pain, [Redacted username], Oneself, Sending, The truth, Quảng Ninh (a Northern province in Vietnam), Bait, Costliness, Heaviness, Jokes, Spa
Topic 30: Aging and loneliness	1.42 (0.23)	Belonging, Myself, Sesame, Animal bones, Chỉ Thống Hoàn (osteoarthritis medication), Cadmium, Diaphoretic, Drawing, Blood, Dr Lê Minh, Viettel (a telecommunication company), Envelope, Shampoo, Ramnoza, Kangaroo, Traditional medicine street, Lipstick, Prescription, Earth, Cat

(continued)

Table A.1: Topics generated and their top 20 terms (continued)

Topic	Share % M (SD)	Top 20 terms (translated)
Topic 31: Old age and health	1.29 (0.39)	Produce, Virus, Grind, Ringworm, Hypertension, Quality, Pleiku (a city in the Central highlands), Food dish, Unit, Coughing, Stew, Everybody, Water pipe, My aunt, Sickness, Manhood, Items★, Pharmacist, [Redacted username], Bad temper
Topic 32: Managing the common cold with TM	2.65 (0.28)	Sky, Capture, Labour, Weight, Panax pseudoginseng, Plant family, Samurai (energy drink brand), Conclusion, [Redacted username], Acyclovir, Buying, Cupping therapy, [Redacted username], The academy, Bravery, Treasure, Majority, Master
Topic 33: Nutrition and cardiovascular health	2.05 (0.19)	Battleground, Soil, Voice, Bran, Tip★, Nun, Quality, Ease, Human organs, Equilibrium, Blood veins, Medical effects, Fruits, Human anatomy, Egg, Cashew, Selection, Alternative, Kidney, Vinegar
Topic 34: Healthy lifestyle and religious narratives	2.02 (0.44)	Winter melon detox juice, Zona, Job's tears seeds, Strawflower tea, Freshness, Observation, Dharmapala, Afternoon, Namo amitabud, Inauguration, The moon★, Fruit, Instance, Beauty, Hibiscus, Medicinality, Multitude, Mint, Adults, Share★
Topic 35: Men's health and cardiovascular health	2.03 (0.60)	Actuality, Chia seeds, Spora Lygodii, Mass communication, Positivity, Magnolia bark, Bracelet, [Redacted username], Flatulence, Sudden, [Redacted username], High endogenous testosterone, Sharing, Total occlusion, Infection, Certainty, Guava, 10kg, Water, Basic
Topic 36: Women's beauty and sexual health	1.02 (0.16)	[Redacted username], Chlorophyll, Helping, Body, Know-how, Soul, Droppers★, Counsellor, Indochinese serrow, [Redacted username], Senior Colonel, Obstetric, Tetronic acid★, Euphorbia ambovombensis, Forrest, North winds, Flabby, Secret code, Ficus★
Topic 37: Narratives of medical families and family recipes	4.01 (1.57)	Efficacy, [Redacted username], False ginseng, Familiy recipe, Household registration book, Goods, Caterpillar fungus powder, Infertility, [Redacted username], Tour★, Retaining, The passing of spring, [Redacted username], Flower, Chickrassy, Water caltrops, Listed price, Wind, Filtered water, Aches, Rice
Topic 38: Insomnia and discussion of burnout	1.37 (0.22)	Disinfection, Wooden floor, Week, Sock★, Burning pain, 'Bread and butter', Year of the Dog, [Redacted username], Virus, Inadequate sleep, Gum, [Redacted username], Jaundice, Root cause, International★, [Redacted username], Caligan★, 330mg, Willow tree, Jelly

Table A.1: Topics generated and their top 20 terms (continued)

Topic	Share % M (SD)	Top 20 terms (translated)
Topic 39: Diet and women's health	3.34 (1.33)	Snake, Forgotten recipes, Multitude, Winged bean pods, Women, Coconut shell, Once upon a time, Waistline, Weight loss, Ignoring, Rice paddy herb, Hypertension, Vestibular disorders, Shellfish, Toxaemia, Đà Nẵng (a city in Central Vietnam), Salt, [Redacted username], Virgin fish sauce
Topic 40: Pregnancy advice	2.94 (0.55)	Gypsum, Choking on a fishbone, Liver, Cornea, Helicteres hirsuta Lour, Long Ju, Flatulence, Aiming, Từ Dũ (an obstetric hospital in Ho Chi Minh City), After-hour shirts, City, Night, Manufacturer, [Redacted username], [Redacted username], Pomade, [Redacted username], Kilogram, Common cold during pregnancy, Legitimacy
Topic 41: Health and beauty tips	2.10 (0.13)	Indian goosegrass, Flower stigma, Someday, Past recipes, Sarsi, Rice paddy herbs, Skills, Member★, Gifting, Blood cockle, Five fruits, Water caltrop, Brother and sisters, Caffeine, Salt, Professional, Delivery, [Redacted username], [Redacted username], Homegrown
Topic 42: Cautionary tales against abuse of indigenous tobacco	1.41 (0.20)	Coronary artery disease, Experience, Thuốc rê (traditional rustic tobacco), [Redacted username], Eggplant, U Minh (commune in Cà Mau, Southernmost province in Vietnam), [Redacted username], Almond, Wisdom teeth, Anticipation, Miracle, Monk fruit, Asthma, Phú Thọ (province in Northern Vietnam), Vestibular disorders, Step, Gấc seeds, Positivity, Origins, Sinusitis
Topic 43: Fantastic tales about the religious and historical origins of Vietnamese medicine	2.73 (0.76)	Miniscule, Today, Baton, Annoyance, Northern Central, Ākāśagarbha (a Buddhist Bodhisattva), Regret, Đà river (Northern Vietnam), The way, [Redacted username], [Redacted username], Himalayas, Needles, Joy, Trưng sisters (ancient history women warriors), Snakehead, Time, Panadol, Accidentality, [Redacted username]
Topic 44: Traditional alternatives to biomedicine and overseas Vietnamese	1.22 (0.19)	Friend, Germany, [Redacted username], Miniscule, Dandruff, Military, Apple, Operation, Nature, Anti-inflammatory, Muscovy duck, Testicles, Timeliness, Heat, Pregnancy, Baby, mmol/L★, Oysters, [Redacted username], Multitude
Topic 45: Constipation and hot/cold binary	4.45 (0.78)	Sickness, Orchid, Loneliness, Orphan, Tightness, Extract, Sharing, Alcohol★, Goose, List, Sapodilla, Hygiene, Remainder, [Redacted username], [Redacted username], [Redacted username], Blue★, Eyedrops, Gulan★, Cooling agent, Purple heart plant

(continued)

Table A.1: Topics generated and their top 20 terms (continued)

Topic	Share % M (SD)	Top 20 terms (translated)
Topic 46: Northern medicine and haemostasis	4.02 (1.09)	Reduction, 50cm, Bleeding, Red beans, Pebbles, Phú Xuyên (a district in Hà Nội), Tip★, Pangolins, Pueraria thomsonii flower extract, Concurrency, Activity, Parasite, Thorns, Cover, Fish, Fungi, Health, Steaming, 1 month, Weighing scale
Topic 47: Nutritions and women's health	3.35 (1.72)	Withdrawal, Overreaction, Name, Mutuality, Aches, Mentality, Jar, Early, Long process, Infection, Sinusitis, Women, Pharmacy, Pouring, Sisters, Soaking, Time, Symptoms, Ming aralia, Crinum latifolium
Topic 48: Pain management with TM	1.78 (0.77)	Raising, Gratitude, Daisy, X-ray, Spinal disc herniation, Hospital, Phoenix eyes, Rambutan, Myself, Dry blood, Gauze, Advice, Cabbage, [Redacted name], Criticism, Quantifying, Superior grade, Poaching, Truthfulness, Sliding
Topic 49: Otolaryngology and TM	1.12 (0.07)	Photograph, Gum, Nose, Care, White, [Redacted username], Cabbage, Bone, Lemon, Buttox, Conclusion, Minority, Life, Bottle cap, Sea, Vitamin B, Children, Papaya, Belching, Hot temper

Note: Terms are translated into English where appropriate. Proper nouns (brand names, location names) are kept in Vietnamese, accompanied by explanations in brackets. Common names of plants are preferred over their scientific names, although not all plants have common names in English. Usernames are redacted to ensure anonymity. Terms that were originally written in a language other than Vietnamese are marked with '★'.

APPENDIX 2

Summary Statistics for the Interpretation of a Topic

Figure A.1: Inter-topic distance map (via multidimensional scaling using the 'LDAvis' package)

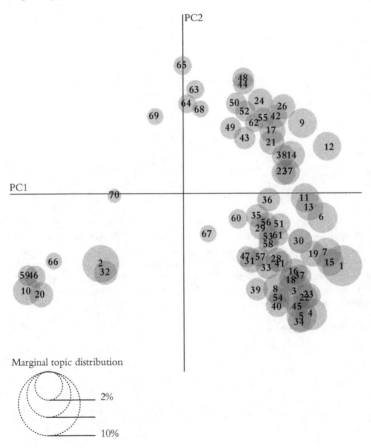

Table A.2: Topic 30: Aging and loneliness

Top words	
$\lambda = 1$	$\lambda = 0.6$
Sesame	Belonging
Animal bones	Myself
Prescription	Sesame
Earth	Animal bones
Belonging	Chỉ Thống Hoàn (osteoarthritis medication)
Dr Lê Minh	Cadmium
Myself	Diaphoretic
Cat	Drawing
Envelope	Blood
Viettel	Dr Lê Minh
Shampoo	Viettel (a telecommunication company)
Chỉ Thống Hoàn (osteoarthritis medication)	Envelope
Diaphoretic	Shampoo
Kangaroo	Ramnoza
Lipstick	Kangaroo
Cadmium	Traditional medicine street
Drawing	Lipstick
Blood	Prescription
Viettel (a telecommunication company)	Earth
Ramnoza	Cat

Note: This statistic presentation is modelled after Maier et al (2018). Figure A.1 depicts a divided table and an inter-topic distance map, where the specific topic in summary is coloured red. Table A.2 maps out the top-words according to two different relevance values ($\lambda = 1$ and $\lambda = .6$). Below the table, the ranks of the Rank-1 and the coherence metrics are given.

Rank-1 metric: rank 37 out of 70

Coherence metric: rank 23 out of 70

Notes

Chapter 2

[1] Georg Simmel (1858–1918) was a German sociologist and neo-Kantian philosopher, best known for his works on sociological methodology. Simmel sought to isolate the general or recurring forms of social interaction from the more specific kinds of activity, such as political, economic, and aesthetic. He also outlined a range of distinctive concepts of contemporary sociology, such as social distance, marginality, urbanism as a way of life, roleplaying, social behaviour as exchange, conflict as an integrating process, dyadic encounter, circular interaction, reference groups as perspectives, and sociological ambivalence.

[2] ANT originated in science studies in the 1980s and became influential in the social sciences more broadly in the late 1990s. ANT is known for its iconoclastic style of argument – a source of inspiration and criticism in equal measures. Ethnomethodologist Michael Lynch (1995, p 168) mockingly suggested that a more appropriate name for ANT might be 'actant-rhizome ontology' – a suggestion that Bruno Latour, in classic ANT fashion, fully embraced. Latour's reservation with this moniker is, however, that it is a 'horrible mouthful of words – not to mention the acronym ARO' (Latour, 1999, p 19).

Chapter 4

[1] Claude E. Shannon (1916–2001), American mathematician, electrical engineer, computer scientist and cryptographer, published an influential article titled 'A mathematical theory of communication' in *Bell System Technical Journal* in 1948, where he formulated what he called 'Printed English', a system consisting of 27 characters – 26 letters of the Latin alphabet plus a character for white space – to enable statistical analysis of the probability that each character would follow a given other.

[2] John von Neumann (1903–57) was a Hungarian-American mathematician, physicist, and computer scientist who is best known for his work in computer architecture. He conceived, raised funds for, and directed the Electronic Computer Project (1945–57) at the Institute for Advanced Study at Princeton, which in 1952 produced one of the first electronic stored-program computers and made significant engineering advances in components and systems design.

References

99firms (2023) 'Facebook Live statistics', Available from: https://99firms. com/blog/facebook-live-stats/#gref [Accessed 8 July 2024].

Agence France-Presse (AFP) (2019, 1 January) 'New year, new repression: Vietnam imposes draconian "China-like" cybersecurity law', *South China Morning Post*, Available from: https://www.scmp.com/news/ asia/southeast-asia/article/2180263/new-year-new-repression-vietnam-imposes-draconian-china [Accessed 8 July 2024].

Albright, J. (2018) 'The Graph API: key points in the Facebook and Cambridge Analytica debacle', *Medium*, Available from: https://medium. com/tow-center/the-graph-api-key-points-in-the-facebook-and-cambri dge-analytica-debacle-b69fe692d747 [Accessed 8 July 2024].

Altheide, D.L. (1995) *An Ecology of Communication: Cultural Formats of Control*, New York: Aldine de Gruyter.

Apprich, C. and Bachmann, G. (2017) 'Media genealogy: back to the present of digital cultures', in G. Koch (ed) *Digitisation: Theories and Concepts for the Empirical Cultural Analysis*, Abingdon: Routledge, pp 293–306.

Armstrong, P.W. and Naylor, C.D. (2019) 'Counteracting health misinformation: a role for medical journals?', *JAMA*, 321(19): 1863–4.

Arun, R., Suresh, V., Madhavan, C.V., and Murthy, M.N. (2010) 'On finding the natural number of topics with latent dirichlet allocation: some observations', in M.J. Zaki, J.X. Yu, B. Ravindran and V. Pud (eds) *Pacific-Asia Conference on Knowledge Discovery and Data Mining*, Berlin, Heidelberg: Springer, pp 391–402.

Association of American Medical Colleges (AAMC) (2023, 28 June) 'Careers in medicine: specialty profiles', Available from: https://careersinmedicine. aamc.org/explore-options/specialty-profiles [Accessed 8 July 2024].

Auslander, P. (2012) 'Digital liveness: a historico-philosophical perspective', *PAJ: A Journal of Performance & Art*, 34(3): 3–11.

Auslander, P., van Es, K., and Hartmann, M. (2019) 'A dialogue about liveness', in M. Hartmann, E. Prommer, K. Decker, and S.O. Gorland (eds) *Mediated Time: Perspectives on Time in a Digital Age*, Cham, Switzerland: Palgrave Macmillan, pp 275–96.

Balachandran, P. and Govindarajan, R. (2005) 'Cancer – an ayurvedic perspective', *Pharmacological Research*, 51(1): 19–30.

Baldanza, K. (2018) 'Publishing, book culture, and reading practices in Vietnam: the view from Thắng Nghiêm and Phổ Nhân Temples', *Journal of Vietnamese Studies*, 13(3): 9–28.

Banerjee, M. (2008) 'Ayurveda in modern India: standardization and pharmaceuticalization', in D. Wujastyk and F.M. Smith (eds) *Modern and Global Ayurveda: Pluralism and Paradigms*, New York: State University of New York Press, pp 201–14.

Bao, Y.X., Wong, C.K., Leung, S.F., Chan, A.T.C., Li, P.W., Wong, E.L.Y. et al (2006) 'Clinical studies of immunomodulatory activities of Yunzhi-Danshen in patients with nasopharyngeal carcinoma', *Journal of Alternative & Complementary Medicine*, 12(8): 771–6.

Bassett, D.S. and Bullmore, E.T. (2017) 'Small-world brain networks revisited', *The Neuroscientist*, 23(5): 499–516.

Bates, D.G. (2000) 'Why not call modern medicine "alternative"?', *Perspectives in Biology & Medicine*, 43(4): 502–18.

Beck, C. (2016) 'Web of resistance: Deleuzian digital space and hacktivism', *Journal for Cultural Research*, 20(4): 334–49.

Bell, S.E. and Figert, A.E. (eds) (2015) *Reimagining (Bio) Medicalization, Pharmaceuticals and Genetics: Old Critiques and New Engagements*, New York: Routledge.

Bent, S. (2008) 'Herbal medicine in the United States: review of efficacy, safety, and regulation', *Journal of General Internal Medicine*, 23(6): 854–9.

Bergson, H. (2002) 'Duration and simultaneity', in K.A. Pearson and J. Mullarkey (eds) *Henri Bergson: Key Writings*, London: Continuum, pp 203–20.

Blei, D.M. (2012) 'Surveying a suite of algorithms that offer a solution to managing large document archives', *Communication of the ACM*, 55(4): 77–84.

Blei, D.M. and Mcauliffe, J. (2007) 'Supervised topic models', Neural Information Processing Systems Proceedings, 21: 121–8.

Blei, D.M., Ng, A.Y., and Jordan, M.I. (2003) 'Latent Dirichlet allocation', *Journal of Machine Learning Research*, 3: 993–1022.

Blok, A. and Pedersen, M.A. (2014) 'Complementary social science? Quali-quantitative experiments in a Big Data world', *Big Data & Society*, 1(2), Available from: https://doi.org/10.1177/2053951714543908 [Accessed 8 July 2024].

Bode, L. and Vraga, E.K. (2018) 'See something, say something: Correction of global health misinformation on social media', *Health Communication*, 33(9): 1131–40.

Bolter, J.D. and Grusin, R. (1999) *Remediation: Understanding New Media*, Cambridge, MA: MIT Press.

Börner, K., Chen, C., and Boyack, K.W. (2003) 'Visualizing knowledge domains', *Annual Review of Information Science & Technology*, 37(1): 179–255.

Broom, A., Doron, A., and Tovey, P. (2009) 'The inequalities of medical pluralism: hierarchies of health, the politics of tradition and the economies of care in Indian oncology', *Social Science & Medicine*, 69(5): 698–706.

Buchanan, I. (2007) 'Deleuze and the internet', *Australian Humanities Review*, 43: 1–19.

Bucher, T. and Helmond, A. (2017) 'The affordances of social media platforms', in J. Burgess, A., Marwock, and T. Poell (eds) *The SAGE Handbook of Social Media*, London: SAGE Publications, pp 233–53.

Caci, B., Cardaci, M., and Tabacchi, M.E. (2012) 'Facebook as a small world: a topological hypothesis', *Social Network Analysis & Mining*, 2(2): 163–7.

Callon, M., Courtial, J.P., and Laville, F. (1991) 'Co-word analysis as a tool for describing the network of interactions between basic and technological research: the case of polymer chemistry', *Scientometrics*, 22(1): 155–205.

Callon, M., Courtial, J.P., Turner, W.A., and Bauin, S. (1983) 'From translations to problematic networks: an introduction to co-word analysis', *Information (International Social Science Council)*, 22(2): 191–235.

Callon, M., Law, J., and Rip, A. (1986) *Mapping the Dynamics of Science and Technology*, Basingstoke, London: The MacMillan Press.

Cao, J., Xia, T., Li, J., Zhang, Y., and Tang, S. (2009) 'A density-based method for adaptive LDA model selection', *Neurocomputing*, 72(7–9): 1775–81.

Carolan, B.V. (2016) 'Social network analysis', *Oxford Bibliographies in Education*, Available from: https://www.oxfordbibliographies.com/display/document/obo-9780199756810/obo-9780199756810-0167.xml [Accessed 8 July 2024].

Caspi, O., Sechrest, L., Pitluk, H.C., and Marshall, C.L. (2003) 'On the definition of complementary, alternative, and integrative medicine: societal mega-stereotypes vs. the patients' perspectives', *Alternative Therapies in Health & Medicine*, 9(6): 58–62.

Cassidy, C.M. (2008) 'Some terminology needs for writers, researchers, practitioners, and editors as we move toward integrating medicines', *Journal of Alternative & Complementary Medicine*, 14(6): 613–15.

Catanese, S.A., De Meo, P., Ferrara, E., Fiumara, G., and Provetti, A. (2011, May) 'Crawling Facebook for social network analysis purposes', in *Proceedings of the International Conference on Web Intelligence, Mining and Semantics*, pp 1–8.

Cerone, A., Naghizade, E., Scholer, F., Mallal, D., Skelton, R., and Spina, D. (2020) 'Watch'n'Check: towards a social media monitoring tool to assist fact-checking experts', in *2020 IEEE 7th International Conference on Data Science and Advanced Analytics (DSAA)*, IEEE, pp 607–13.

Chandran, S. (2020, 30 March) '#MYStayHome: More demand for traditional herbs to boost immunity during Covid-19', *The Star*, Available from: https://www.thestar.com.my/lifestyle/living/2020/03/30/mystayh ome-beeline-for-traditional-herbs-to-boost-immunity-during-covid-19 [Accessed 8 July 2024].

Chou, W.Y.S., Oh, A., and Klein, W.M. (2018) 'Addressing health-related misinformation on social media', *JAMA*, 320(23): 2417–18.

Chung, H.J. (2018) *Media Heterotopias: Digital Effects and Material Labor in Global Film Production*, Durham, NC: Duke University Press.

Corrales-Garay, D., Ortiz-de-Urbina-Criado, M., and Mora-Valentín, E.M. (2019) 'Knowledge areas, themes and future research on open data: a co-word analysis', *Government Information Quarterly*, 36(1): 77–87.

Craig, D. (2002) *Familiar Medicine: Everyday Health Knowledge and Practice in Today's Vietnam*, Honolulu, HI: University of Hawaii Press.

Csardi, G. and Nepusz, T. (2006) 'The igraph software package for complex network research', *InterJournal, Complex Systems*, 1695(5): 1–9.

Daston, L. and Galison, P. (2007) *Objectivity*, New York: Zone Books.

Davis, J.L. (2020) *How Artifacts Afford: The Power and Politics of Everyday Things*, Cambridge, MA: MIT Press.

de Vries, L. (2022) 'Vietnam in the pre-modern period', in V. Lo, D. Yang, and M. Stanley-Baker (eds) *Routledge Handbook of Chinese Medicine*, London, New York: Routledge, pp 493–502.

DeFrancis, J. (1977) *Colonialism and Language Policy in Viet Nam*, The Hague: Mouton Publishers.

DiMaggio, P. (2015) 'Adapting computational text analysis to social science (and vice versa)', *Big Data & Society*, 2(2): 1–5.

Dong, H., Bogg, L., Rehnberg, C., and Diwan, V. (1999) 'Drug policy in China: pharmaceutical distribution in rural areas', *Social Science & Medicine*, 48(6): 777–86.

Drucker, J. (2001) 'Digital ontologies: the ideality of form in/and code storage – or – can graphesis challenge mathesis?' *Leonardo*, 34(2): 141–5.

Elsevier (2023, 28 June) 'Scopus content coverage guide', Available from: https://assets.ctfassets.net/o78em1y1w4i4/EX1iy8VxBeQKf8aN2XzOp/ c36f79db25484cb38a5972ad9a5472ec/Scopus_ContentCoverage_Guide_ WEB.pdf [Accessed 8 July 2024].

Epskamp, S., Costantini, G., Haslbeck, J., Cramer, A.O., Waldorp, L.J., Schmittmann, V.D. et al (2019) 'Package "qgraph"', Available from: https:// cran.r-project.org/web/packages/qgraph/qgraph.pdf [Accessed 8 July 2024].

Erikson, E. (2013) 'Formalist and relationalist theory in social network analysis', *Sociological Theory*, 31(3): 219–42.

Ernst, E. (1998) 'Chiropractors' use of X-rays', *British Journal of Radiology*, 71(843): 249–51.

Ettlinger, N. (2018) 'Algorithmic affordances for productive resistance', *Big Data & Society*, 5(1), Available from: https://doi.org/10.1177/205395171 8771399 [Accessed 8 July 2024].

Evans, M.S. (2014) 'A computational approach to qualitative analysis in largetextual datasets', *PloS One*, 9(2): e87908. 10.1371/journal. pone.0087908

Facebook (2021, 26 July) 'Terms of service', Available from: https://www. facebook.com/legal/terms/plain_text_terms [Accessed 8 July 2024].

Flis, I. and van Eck, N.J. (2018) 'Framing psychology as a discipline (1950–1999): a large-scale term co-occurrence analysis of scientific literature in psychology', *History of Psychology*, 21(4): 334–62.

Fobar, R. (2020, 26 March) 'China promotes bear bile as coronavirus treatment, alarming wildlife advocates', *National Geographic*, Available from: https://www.nationalgeographic.com/animals/article/chinese-gov ernment-promotes-bear-bile-as-coronavirus-covid19-treatment#close [Accessed 8 July 2024].

Foucault, M. (1963) *The Birth of the Clinic*, London, New York: Routledge.

Foucault, M. (1966) *The Order of Things*, London, New York: Routledge.

Foucault, M. (1977) *Discipline and Punish: The Birth of the Prison*, London, New York: Penguin.

Foucault, M. (1984, October) 'Des Espace Autres' [Of other spaces: utopias and heterotopias], *Architecture/Mouvement/Continuité*, 5: 46–9, translated by J. Miskowiec, Available from: https://web.mit.edu/allanmc/www/foucau lt1.pdf [Accessed 8 July 2024].

Franklin, S. (2015) *Control: Digitality as Cultural Logic*, Cambridge, MA: MIT Press.

Frey, B. (2018) *The SAGE Encyclopedia of Educational Research, Measurement, and Evaluation* (Vols 1–4), Thousand Oaks, CA: SAGE Publications.

Fuller, M. (2007) *Media Ecologies: Materialist Energies in Art and Technoculture*, Cambridge, MA: MIT Press.

Gale, N. (2014) 'The sociology of traditional, complementary and alternative medicine', *Sociology Compass*, 8(6): 805–22.

Galloway, A.R. (2014) *Laruelle: Against the Digital*, Minneapolis, MN: University of Minnesota Press.

Gan, N. and Xiong, Y. (2020, 16 March) 'Beijing is promoting traditional medicine as a "Chinese solution" to coronavirus. Not everyone is on board', *CNN*, Available from: https://edition.cnn.com/2020/03/14/asia/ coronavirus-traditional-chinese-medicine-intl-hnk/index.html [Accessed 8 July 2024].

Gell, A. (1988) 'Technology and magic', *Anthropology Today*, 4(2): 6–9.

General Medical Council (GMC) (2023, 28 June) 'GMC approved postgraduate curricula', Available from: https://www.gmc-uk.org/educat ion/standards-guidance-and-curricula/curricula [Accessed 8 July 2024].

Gerlach, M., Peixoto, T.P., and Altmann, E.G. (2018) 'A network approach to topic models', *Science Advances*, 4(7): eaaq1360.

Ghenai, A. and Mejova, Y. (2018) 'Fake cures: user-centric modeling of health misinformation in social media', *Proceedings of the ACM on Human–Computer Interaction*, 2(CSCW): 1–20.

Graham, M. (2013) 'Geography/internet: ethereal alternate dimensions of cyberspace or grounded augmented realities?' *The Geographical Journal* 179(2): 177–82.

Graham, T. and Ackland, R. (2016) 'SocialMediaLab: tools for collecting social media data and generating networks for analysis', CRAN (The Comprehensive R Archive Network), Available from: https://cran.rproject.org/web/packages/SocialMediaLab/SocialMediaLab.pdf [Accessed 8 July 2024].

Griffin, M., Herrmann, S., and Kittler, F.A. (1996) 'Technologies of writing: interview with Friedrich A. Kittler', *New Literary History*, 27(4): 731–42.

Griffiths, T.L. and Steyvers, M. (2004) 'Finding scientific topics', *Proceedings of the National Academy of Sciences*, 101(Suppl. 1): 5228–35.

Grün, B. and Hornik, K. (2011) 'Topicmodels: an R package for fitting topic models', *Journal of Statistical Software*, 40(13): 1–30.

Guy, J.S. (2018) 'Is Niklas Luhmann a relational sociologist?' in F. Dépelteau (ed) *The Palgrave Handbook of Relational Sociology*, Cham, Switzerland: Palgrave Macmillan, pp 289–304.

Halappanavar, S., Vogel, U., Wallin, H., and Yauk, C.L. (2018) 'Promise and peril in nanomedicine: the challenges and needs for integrated systems biology approaches to define health risk', *Wiley Interdisciplinary Reviews: Nanomedicine & Nanobiotechnology*, 10(1): 14–65.

Han, G.S. and Ballis, H. (2007) 'Ethnomedicine and dominant medicine in multicultural Australia: a critical realist reflection on the case of Korean-Australian immigrants in Sydney', *Journal of Ethnobiology & Ethnomedicine*, 3(1): 1.

Hanckel, B., Vivienne, S., Byron, P., Robards, B., and Churchill, B. (2019) '"That's not necessarily for them": LGBTIQ+ young people, social media platform affordances and identity curation', *Media, Culture & Society*, 41(8): 1261–78.

Hannas, W.C. (1997) *Asia's Orthographic Dilemma*, Honolulu, HI: University of Hawaii Press.

Hanneman, R.A. and Riddle, M. (2016) 'Concepts and measures for basic network analysis', in J. Scott and P.J. Carrington (eds) *The SAGE Handbook of Social Network Analysis*, EBook Central, ProQuest, pp 340–68.

Hansen, M.B. (2015) *Feed-Forward: On the Future of Twenty-First-Century Media*, Chicago, IL: University of Chicago Press.

Hanson, M. (2011) *Speaking of Epidemics in Chinese Medicine: Disease and the Geographic Imagination in Late Imperial China*, London, New York: Routledge.

Haraway, D. (1988) 'Situated knowledges: the science question in feminism and the privilege of partial perspective', *Feminist Studies*, 14(3): 575–99.

Harrington, A. (2008) *The Cure Within: A History of Mind-Body Medicine*, New York, London, W.W. Norton & Co.

Hassan, R. (2011) *The Age of Distraction: Reading, Writing, and Politics in a High-Speed Networked Economy*, London: Transaction Publishers.

Hayles, N.K. (2004) 'Print is flat, code is deep: the importance of media-specific analysis', *Poetics Today*, 25(1): 67–90.

He, Q. (1999) 'Knowledge discovery through co-word analysis', *Library Trends*, 48(1): 133–59.

Hess, A. (2008) 'Reconsidering the rhizome: a textual analysis of web search engines as gatekeepers of the internet', in A. Spink and M. Zimmer (eds) *Web Search: Multidisciplinary Perspectives*, Berlin, Heidelberg: Springer, pp 35–50.

Hether, H.J., Murphy, S.T., and Valente, T.W. (2016) 'A social network analysis of supportive interactions on prenatal sites', *Digital Health*, 2: 1–12.

Hirsch Jr, E.D. (1977) *The Philosophy of Composition*, Chicago, IL: University of Chicago Press.

Hoang, T.A. (2015) 'Modelling user interest and community interest in microbloggings: an integrated approach', in T. Cao, E.-P. Lim, Z.-H. Zhou, T.-B. Ho, D. Cheung and H. Motoda (eds) *Pacific-Asia Conference on Knowledge Discovery and Data Mining*, Cham, Switzerland: Springer, pp 708–21.

Hobsbawm, E. and Ranger, T. (eds) (2012) *The Invention of Tradition*, Cambridge: Cambridge University Press.

Hodgkin, T. (1981) *Vietnam: The Revolutionary Path*, London: Macmillan Press.

Hoi Dong, Y. (2019, 4 June) 'Overview of Vietnam Association of Traditional Medicine', Available from: https://hoidongy.vn/category/gioi-thieu/gioi-thieu-gioi-thieu/ [Accessed 30 August 2024].

Hou-Liu, J. (2018) 'Benchmarking and improving recovery of number of topics in latent Dirichlet allocation models', Available from: https://pdfs.semanticscholar.org/2175/aa77463e23da96281cc2fb5125e0b9de3bbd.pdf [Accessed 8 July 2024].

Huhtamo, E. and Parikka, J. (2011) *Media Archaeology: Approaches, Applications, and Implications*, Oakland, CA: University of California Press.

Humphries, M.D. and Gurney, K. (2008) 'Network "small-world-ness": a quantitative method for determining canonical network equivalence', *PLoS One*, 3(4): e0002051.

Huong Thu (2022, 15 August) 'Vietnam Southern Medicine Association changes its name to Vietnam Traditional Medicine Association', *Tuổi Trẻ Thủ Đô*, Available from: https://tuoitrethudo.com.vn/hoi-nam-y-viet-nam-doi-ten-thanh-hoi-y-duoc-co-truyen-viet-nam-205828.html [Accessed 30 August 2024].

Hwang, T. (2020) 'Deconstructing the disinformation war', *MediaWell*, Available from: https://mediawell.ssrc.org/expert-reflections/deconstructing-the-disinformation-war/ [Accessed 8 July 2024].

Igami, M.P.Z., Bressiani, J.C., and Mugnaini, R. (2014) 'A new model to identify the productivity of theses in terms of articles using co-word analysis', *Journal of Scientometric Research*, 3(1): 3.

Internet World Stats (2023) 'Internet 2022 usage in Asia', Available from: https://www.internetworldstats.com/stats3.htm [Accessed 8 July 2024].

Jones, L. (2018) *Haptics*, Cambridge, MA: MIT Press.

Juhlin, O., Engström, A., and Reponen, E. (2010) 'Mobile broadcasting', in *Proceedings of the 12th International Conference on Human Computer Interaction with Mobile Devices and Services*, Lisbon, 7–10 September, pp 35–44.

Juneja, P. and Mitra, T. (2022) 'Human and technological infrastructures of fact-checking', *Proceedings of the ACM on Human-Computer Interaction*, 6(CSCW2): 1–36.

Kaptchuk, T.J. and Eisenberg, D.M. (2001) 'Varieties of healing: a taxonomy of unconventional healing practices', *Annals of Internal Medicine*, 135(3): 196–204.

Karpozilos, A. and Pavlidis, N. (2004) 'The treatment of cancer in Greek antiquity', *European Journal of Cancer*, 40(14): 2033–40.

Kemp, S. (2023, 13 February) 'Digital 2023: Vietnam', *DataReportal*, Available from: https://datareportal.com/reports/digital-2023-vietnam [Accessed 8 July 2024].

Kittler, F. (1996) 'The history of communication media', *CTheory*, 7–30.

Laaksonen, S.M., Nelimarkka, M., Tuokko, M., Marttila, M., Kekkonen, A., and Villi, M. (2017) 'Working the fields of big data: using big-data-augmented online ethnography to study candidate–candidate interaction at election time', *Journal of Information Technology & Politics*, 14(2): 110–31.

Lambert, H. (2012) 'Medical pluralism and medical marginality: bone doctors and the selective legitimation of therapeutic expertise in India', *Social Science & Medicine*, 74(7): 1029–36.

Lambert, H. (2018) 'Indian therapeutic hierarchies and the politics of recognition', *Asian Medicine*, 13(1–2): 115–33.

Latour, B. (1988) *Science in Action: How to Follow Scientists and Engineers through Society*, Cambridge, MA: Harvard University Press.

Latour, B. (1993) *The Pasteurization of France*, Cambridge, MA: Harvard University Press.

Latour, B. (1999) 'On recalling ANT', in J. Law and J. Hassard (eds) *Actor-Network Theory and After*, Oxford: Blackwell, pp 15–25.

Latour, B. (2005) *Reassembling the Social: An Introduction to Actor-Network-Theory*, Oxford: Oxford University Press.

Latour, B. and Woolgar, S. (1979) *Laboratory Life: The Construction of Scientific Facts*, Beverley Hills, CA: SAGE Publications.

Latour, B. and Woolgar, S. (1986) *Laboratory Life*, Princeton, NJ: Princeton University Press.

Latour, B., Mauguin, P., and Teil, G. (1992) 'A note on socio-technical graphs', *Social Studies of Science*, 22(1): 33–57.

Latour, B., Jensen, P., Venturini, T., Grauwin, S., and Boullier, D. (2012) '"The whole is always smaller than its parts": a digital test of Gabriel Tardes' monads', *British Journal of Sociology*, 63(4): 590–615.

Law, J. and Mol, A. (1995) 'Notes on materiality and sociality', *The Sociological Review*, 43(2): 274–94.

Le, H.P., Nguyen, T.M.H., Roussanaly, A., and Ho, T.V. (2008) 'A hybrid approach to word segmentation of Vietnamese texts', in C. Martín-Vide, F. Otto and H. Fernau (eds) *Proceedings of the 2nd International Conference on Language and Automata Theory and Applications*, pp 240–9.

Leung, P.C., Ooi, V., Wong, E.L.Y., Au, W.C., Wong, C.K., Lam, W.K. et al (2007) 'Chinese medicine and cancer treatment in Hong Kong: a general review', in P.C. Leung and H. Fong (eds) *Alternative Treatment for Cancer*, Singapore: World Scientific Publishing, pp 65–76.

Li, J. (2020) 'Toward a research agenda on political misinformation and corrective information', *Political Communication*, 37(1): 125–35.

Li, P.W. (1996) *Clinical Oncology for Chinese and Western Practitioners*, Beijing: China Press of Traditional Medicine.

Liebeskind, C. and Liebeskind, S. (2018) 'Identifying abusive comments in Hebrew Facebook', in *2018 IEEE International Conference on the Science of Electrical Engineering in Israel* (ICSEE), IEEE, pp 1–5.

Lim, G.Y. (2020, 11 March) 'Coconut and COVID-19: Philippines studying antiviral properties of coconut oil as potential treatment', *Nutra-Ingredients Asia*, Available from: https://www.nutraingredients-asia.com/Article/2020/03/11/Coconut-and-COVID-19-Philippines-studying-antiviral-properties-of-coconut-oil-as-potential-treatment [Accessed 8 July 2024].

Lindquist, R., Tracy, M.F., and Snyder, M. (eds) (2018) *Complementary & Alternative Therapies in Nursing* (8th edn), New York: Springer.

Lobinger, K. (2016) 'Photographs as things – photographs of things: a texto-material perspective on photo-sharing practices', *Information, Communication & Society*, 19(4): 475–88.

Lock, M. and Nguyen, V.K. (2010) *An Anthropology of Biomedicine*, Chichester: John Wiley & Sons.

Lovink, G. (2011) 'My first recession: critical internet culture in transition', *Institute of Network Cultures*, Available from: https://doi.org/10.25969/mediarep/19271 [Accessed 8 July 2024].

Löwy, I. (2011) 'Historiography of biomedicine: "bio", "medicine", and in between', *Isis*, 102(1): 116–22.

Lu, X., Yu, Z., Guo, B., and Zhou, X. (2014) 'Predicting the content dissemination trends by repost behavior modelling in mobile social networks', *Journal of Network & Computer Applications*, 42: 197–207.

Lury, C. (2012) '"Bringing the world into the world": The material semiotics of contemporary culture', *Distinktion: Scandinavian Journal of Social Theory*, 13(3): 247–60.

Lury, C. (2021) *Problem Spaces: How and Why Methodology Matters*, Chichester: John Wiley & Sons.

Lv, Y., Ding, Y., Song, M., and Duan, Z. (2018) 'Topology-driven trend analysis for drug discovery', *Journal of Informetrics*, 12(3): 893–905.

Lynch, M. (1995) 'Building a global infrastructure', *Studies in History & Philosophy of Science*, 26(1): 167–72.

Ma, S., Zhang, C., and He, D. (2016) 'Document representation methods for clustering bilingual documents', in *Proceedings of the 79th ASIS&T Annual Meeting: Creating Knowledge, Enhancing Lives through Information & Technology*, American Society for Information Science, p 65.

Mackenzie, A. and Munster, A. (2019) 'Platform seeing: image ensembles and their invisualities', *Theory, Culture & Society*, 36(5): 3–22.

Maier, D., Waldherr, A., Miltner, P., Wiedemann, G., Niekler, A., Keinert, A. et al (2018) 'Applying LDA topic modelling in communication research: toward a valid and reliable methodology', *Communication Methods & Measures*, 12(2–3): 93–118.

Malpas, J. (2018) *Place and Experience: A Philosophical Topography*, London, New York: Routledge.

Marin, A. and Wellman, B. (2011) 'Social network analysis: an introduction', in J. Scott and P.J. Carrington (eds) *The SAGE Handbook of Social Network Analysis*, London: SAGE Publications, pp 11–25.

Marr, D. (1987) 'Vietnamese attitudes regarding illness and healing', in N.G. Owen (ed) *Death and Disease in Southeast Asia: Explorations in Social, Medical and Demographic History*, Oxford: Oxford University Press, pp 162–86.

McGann, J. (2016) *Radiant Textuality: Literary Studies after the World Wide Web*, Basingstoke, New York: Springer.

Medical Board of Australia (MBA) (2018, 1 June) 'Medical specialties and specialty fields', Available from: https://www.medicalboard.gov.au/regis tration/types/specialist-registration/medical-specialties-and-specialty-fie lds.aspx [Accessed 8 July 2024].

Meyer, E.T. and Schroeder, R. (2009) 'Untangling the web of e-Research: towards a sociology of online knowledge', *Journal of Informetrics*, 3(3): 246–60.

Meyersohn, N. (2020, 3 March) 'Americans are panic shopping for hand sanitizer and face masks', *CNN*, Available from: https://edition.cnn.com/ 2020/03/03/business/panic-buying-coronavirus-retail-shopping/index. html [Accessed 8 July 2024].

MIC (2023) 'Report on internet statistics of Vietnam', Available from: https://thongkeinternet.vn/jsp/trangchu/index.jsp [Accessed 30 August 2024].

Michael, M. (2017) *Actor-Network Theory: Trials, Trails and Translations*, London: SAGE Publications.

Mimno, D., Wallach, H., Talley, E., Leenders, M., and McCallum, A. (2011, July) 'Optimizing semantic coherence in topic models', in *Proceedings of the 2011 Conference on Empirical Methods in Natural Language Processing*, pp 262–72.

Minh, H. (2018, 28 December) 'Overseas remittances to Vietnam continue increasing', *Sai Gon Giai Phong News Online*, Available from: https://m.sggpnews.org.vn/business/overseas-remittances-to-vietnam-continue-increasing-79438.html [Accessed 8 July 2024].

Moats, D. (2021) 'Rethinking the "great divide": approaching interdisciplinary collaborations around digital data with humour and irony', *Science & Technology Studies*, 34(1): 19–42.

Mol, A. (2002) *The Body Multiple*, Durham, NC: Duke University Press.

Mol, A. (2008) *The Logic of Care: Health and the Problem of Patient Choice*, London: Routledge.

Monnais, L. (2019) *The Colonial Life of Pharmaceuticals*, Cambridge: Cambridge University Press.

Monnais, L. and Tousignant, N. (2006) 'The colonial life of pharmaceuticals: accessibility to healthcare, consumption of medicines, and medical pluralism in French Vietnam, 1905–1945', *Journal of Vietnamese Studies*, 1(1–2): 131–66.

Monnais, L., Thompson, C.M., and Wahlberg, A. (2011) *Southern Medicine for Southern People: Vietnamese Medicine in the Making*, Cambridge: Cambridge Scholars Publishing.

Morita, A. (2020) 'Can ANT compare with anthropology?' In A. Blok, I. Farías, and C. Roberts (eds) *The Routledge Companion to Actor-Network Theory*, London: Routledge, pp 34–45.

Munk, A.K. (2019) 'Four styles of quali-quantitative analysis: making sense of the new Nordic food movement on the web', *Nordicom Review*, 40(1): 159–76.

Murphy, L.S., Reinsch, S., Najm, W.I., Dickerson, V.M., Seffinger, M.A., Adams, A. et al (2003) 'Searching biomedical databases on complementary medicine: the use of controlled vocabulary among authors, indexers and investigators', *BMC Complementary & Alternative Medicine*, 3(1): 3.

Napolitano, V. and Mora Flores, G. (2003) 'Complementary medicine: cosmopolitan and popular knowledge, and transcultural translations-cases from urban Mexico', *Theory, Culture & Society*, 20(4): 79–95.

Nedelcu, M. (2019) 'Digital diasporas', in R. Cohen and C. Fischer (eds) *Routledge Handbook of Diaspora Studies*, London, New York: Routledge, pp 241–50.

Newman, M.E. (2009) 'Random graphs with clustering', *Physical Review Letters*, 103(5): 058701.

Newman, M.E., Moore, C., and Watts, D.J. (2000) 'Mean-field solution of the small-world network model', *Physical Review Letters*, 84(14): 3201.

Nguyen, D. (2020, 24 April) 'Traditional medicine and quest for Covid-19 cure', *Yale Global Online*, Available from: https://archive-yaleglobal.yale.edu/content/traditional-medicine-and-quest-covid-19-cure [Accessed 8 July 2024].

Nguyen, D. (2021a) 'Can't wait to feel better: Facebook Live and the recalibration of downtime in tending to the body', *Media, Culture & Society*, 43(6): 984–99.

Nguyen, D. (2021b) 'Dropping in, helping out: social support and weak ties on traditional medicine social networking sites', *Howard Journal of Communications*, 32(3): 235–52.

Nguyen, T.C., Pham, V.T., and Nguyen, V.T. (2018) 'Buddhist print culture in nineteenth-century Northern Vietnam: a case study of the woodblock collection in Khê Hồi Temple', *Journal of Vietnamese Studies*, 13(3): 51–87.

Nigenda, G., Lockett, L., Manca, C., and Mora, G. (2001) 'Non-biomedical health care practices in the State of Morelos, Mexico: analysis of an emergent phenomenon', *Sociology of Health & Illness*, 23(1): 3–23.

Nikita, M. (2016) 'Package "idatuning": tuning of the latent Dirichlet allocation models parameters', r package version 1.0.0, Available from: https://cran.r-project.org/web/packages/ldatuning/ldatuning.pdf [Accessed 8 July 2024].

Nowotny, H. (1989) *Eigenzeit: Entstehung und strukturierung eines zeitgefühls*, Frankfurt am Main: Suhrkamp.

Nowotny, H. (2019) 'Eigenzeit. Revisited', in M. Hartmann, E. Prommer, K. Decker, and S.O. Gorland (eds) *Mediated Time: Perspectives on Time in a Digital Age*, Cham, Switzerland: Palgrave Macmillan, pp 67–85.

Nunziato, D.C. (2020) 'Misinformation mayhem: social media platforms' efforts to combat medical and political misinformation', *First Amendment Law Review*, 19: 32.

Oeldorf-Hirsch, A. and Sundar, S.S. (2016) 'Social and technological motivations for online photo sharing', *Journal of Broadcasting & Electronic Media*, 60(4): 624–42.

Ogle, B.M., Tuyet, H.T., Duyet, H.N., and Dung, N.N.X. (2003) 'Food, feed or medicine: the multiple functions of edible wild plants in Vietnam', *Economic Botany*, 57(1): 103–17.

Olson, D.R. (1980) 'On the language and authority of textbooks', *Journal of Communication*, 30(1): 186–96.

Olson, E.A. (2016) 'Using plants as medicines and health foods in southern Jalisco', in E.A. Olson and J.R. Stepp (eds) *Plants and Health: New Perspectives on the Health-Environment-Plant Nexus*, Cham, Switzerland: Springer, pp 117–31.

Ong, W.J. (2002) *Orality and Literacy*, Routledge.

Online Newspaper of the Government (2012, 24 April) 'Vietnam is among five most advanced countries in acupuncture', *Online Newspaper of the Government*, Available from: http://baochinhphu.vn/Khoa-hoc-Cong-nghe/Viet-Nam-la-1-trong-5-nuoc-co-nganh-cham-cuu-tien-tien-nhat/136160.vgp [Accessed 8 July 2024].

OpenNet Initiative (2012) 'Region: Asia', Available from: https://opennet.net/research/regions/asia [Accessed 8 July 2024].

Opsahl, T., Vernet, A., Alnuaimi, T., and George, G. (2017) 'Revisiting the small-world phenomenon: efficiency variation and classification of small-world networks', *Organizational Research Methods*, 20(1): 149–73.

Pashigian, M. (2012) 'East, west, north, south: medical pluralism and "suitable" medicine for infertility in contemporary Vietnam', in L. Monnais, M. Thompson, and A. Wahlberg (eds) *Southern Medicine for Southern People: Vietnamese Medicine in the Making*, Cambridge: Cambridge Scholar Publishing, pp 203–26.

Paul, M.J. and Dredze, M. (2012) 'A model for mining public health topics from Twitter', *Health*, 11(16): 1.

Phu Nu Viet Nam (2022, 16 September) 'Introducing the Vietnam Traditional Medicine Association', *Phu Nu Viet Nam*, Available from: https://phunuvietnam.vn/ra-mat-hoi-y-hoc-co-truyen-viet-nam-20220916061210067.htm [Accessed 8 July 2024].

Pieroni, A. and Price, L. (2006) *Eating and Healing: Traditional Food as Medicine*, Binghamton, NY: CRC Press.

Raman A., Tyson G., and Sastry N. (2018, April) Facebook (A) Live? Are live social broadcasts really broadcasts?' in *Proceedings of the 2018 World Wide Web Conference*, pp 1491–500.

Ramati, I. and Pinchevski, A. (2018) 'Uniform multilingualism: a media genealogy of Google Translate', *New Media & Society*, 20(7): 2550–65.

Ravikumar, S., Agrahari, A., and Singh, S.N. (2015) 'Mapping the intellectual structure of scientometrics: a co-word analysis of the journal Scientometrics (2005–2010)', *Scientometrics*, 102(1): 929–55.

Rein, K. and Venturini, T. (2018) 'Ploughing digital landscapes: how Facebook influences the evolution of live video streaming', *New Media & Society*, 20(9): 3359–80.

Ríssola, E.A., Bahrainian, S.A., and Crestani, F. (2019) 'Anticipating Depression Based on Online Social Media Behaviour', in *International Conference on Flexible Query Answering Systems*, Cham, Switzerland: Springer, pp 278–90.

Rogers, R. and Marres, N. (2000) 'Landscaping climate change: a mapping technique for understanding science and technology debates on the World Wide Web', *Public Understanding of Science*, 9(2): 141–63.

Ronda-Pupo, G.A. and Guerras-Martin, L.Á. (2012) 'Dynamics of the evolution of the strategy concept 1962–2008: a co-word analysis', *Strategic Management Journal*, 33(2): 162–88.

Rose, N. (2007) 'Beyond medicalisation', *The Lancet*, 369(9562): 700–2.

Ruckenstein, M. (2019) 'Tracing medicinal agencies: antidepressants and life-effects', *Social Science & Medicine*, 235: 112368.

Rymarczuk, R. and Derksen, M. (2014) 'Different spaces: exploring Facebook as heterotopia', *First Monday*, 19(6): 1–11.

Sai Gon Giai Phong (2012a) 'The hazy truth behind the dien chan method, part 1: telling the real from the fake', *Sai Gon Giai Phong Online*, Available from: https://www.sggp.org.vn/mo-ho-lieu-phap-dien-chan-bai-1-thuc-hu-dien-chan-130343.html [Accessed 8 July 2024].

Sai Gon Giai Phong (2012b) 'The hazy truth behind the dien chan method, part 2: unproven efficacy', *Sai Gon Giai Phong Online*. Available from: http://www.sggp.org.vn/mo-ho-lieu-phap-dien-chan-bai-2-hieu-qua-chua-duoc-minh-dinh-130407.html [Accessed 8 July 2024].

Sai Gon Giai Phong (2012c) 'A follow up on the dien chan method: legal actions will be taken on unauthorized medical treatments', *Sai Gon Giai Phong Online*, Available from: https://www.sggp.org.vn/phan-hoi-tu-bai-viet-mo-ho-lieu-phap-dien-chan-se-xu-ly-viec-kham-chua-benh-trai-phep-130463.html [Accessed 8 July 2024].

Salguero, C. (2018) 'Buddhist medicine and its circulation', in *Oxford Research Encyclopedia of Asian History*, Available from: https://oxfordre.com/asianhist ory/view/10.1093/acrefore/9780190277727.001.0001/acrefore-978019 0277727-e-215 [Accessed 8 July 2024].

Scheid, V. (2002) *Chinese Medicine in Contemporary China: Plurality and Synthesis*, Durham, NC: Duke University Press.

Scheid, V. (2007) *Currents of Tradition in Chinese Medicine, 1626–2006*, Seattle, WA: Eastland Press.

Schillmeier, M. (2014) *Eventful Bodies: The Cosmopolitics of Illness*, Farnham, UK: Ashgate.

Sherman, J. (2019, 11 December) 'Vietnam's Internet Control: Following in China's Footsteps?', *The Diplomat*, Available from: https://thediplomat.com/2019/12/vietnams-internet-control-following-in-chinas-footsteps/ [Accessed 8 July 2024].

Shorofi, S.A. and Arbon, P. (2017) 'Complementary and alternative medicine (CAM) among Australian hospital-based nurses: knowledge, attitude, personal and professional use, reasons for use, CAM referrals, and socio-demographic predictors of CAM users', *Complementary Therapies in Clinical Practice*, 27: 37–45.

Sievert, C. and Shirley, K. (2014, June) 'LDAvis: a method for visualizing and interpreting topics', in *Proceedings of the Workshop on Interactive Language Learning, Visualization, and Interfaces*, pp 63–70. 10.3115/v1/W14-3110

Smith, N. and Graham, T. (2019) 'Mapping the anti-vaccination movement on Facebook', *Information, Communication & Society*, 22(9): 1310–27.

Statt, N. (2019, 1 May) 'Facebook is redesigning its core app around the two parts people actually like to use', *The Verge*, Available from: https://www.theverge.com/2019/4/30/18523265/facebook-events-groups-redesign-news-feed-features-f8-2019 [Accessed 8 July 2024].

Stegmann, J. and Grohmann, G. (2003) 'Hypothesis generation guided by co-word clustering', *Scientometrics*, 56(1): 111–35.

Steiner, P. (1993, 5 July) 'On the internet, nobody knows you're a dog' [cartoon], *The New Yorker* 69(LXIX): 61.

Stratton, J. (2021) 'Coronavirus, the great toilet paper panic and civilisation', *Thesis Eleven*, 165(1): 145–68.

Suc Khoe Doi Song (2022, 25 October) 'Người được mệnh danh là "ông tổ" thuốc Nam và mở đầu cho nền y dược cổ truyền của Việt Nam' [The grandfather of Southern medicine and pioneer for Vietnamese traditional medicine], *Suc Khoe Doi Song Online*, Available at: https://suckhoedoisong.vn/nguoi-duoc-menh-danh-la-ong-to-thuoc-nam-va-mo-dau-cho-nen-y-duoc-co-truyen-cua-viet-nam-169221025151948931.htm [Accessed 8 July 2024].

Sudhakar, A. (2009) 'History of cancer, ancient and modern treatment methods', *Journal of Cancer Science & Therapy*, 1(2): 1.

Swire, B., Berinsky, A.J., Lewandowsky, S., and Ecker, U.K. (2017) 'Processing political misinformation: comprehending the Trump phenomenon', *Royal Society Open Science*, 4(3): 160802.

Taylor, C.E. (1976) 'The place of indigenous medical practitioners in the modernization of health services', in C. Leslie (ed) *Asian Medical Systems: A Comparative Study*, Berkeley, CA: University of California Press, pp 285–99.

Telesford, Q.K., Joyce, K.E., Hayasaka, S., Burdette, J.H., and Laurienti, P.J. (2011) 'The ubiquity of small-world networks', *Brain Connectivity*, 1(5): 367–75.

Templeman, K., Robinson, A., and McKenna, L. (2015) 'Student identification of the need for complementary medicine education in Australian medical curricula: a constructivist grounded theory approach', *Complementary Therapies in Medicine*, 23(2): 257–64.

Tenen, D. (2017) *Plain Text: The Poetics of Computation*, Redwood City, CA: Stanford University Press.

Thang, D.Q., Phuong, L.H., Huyen, N.T.M., Tu, N.C., Rossignol, M., and Luong, V.X. (2008) 'Word segmentation of Vietnamese texts: a comparison of approaches', in *Proceedings of the 6th International Conference on Language Resources and Evaluation*, pp 1933–6.

That Son (2016, 24 March) 'Đấu giá sách hiếm ở "Không gian sách cũ" tại Hà Nội' [Rare book auction at 'Old book space' in Hanoi], *VNExpress*, Available from: https://vnexpress.net/dau-gia-sach-hiem-o-khong-gian-sach-cu-tai-ha-noi-3375318.html [Accessed 8 July 2024].

The Nation Thailand (2020, 21 February) 'The plant that might stop Covid-19', *The Nation Thailand*, Available from: https://www.nationthail and.com/news/30382571 [Accessed 8 July 2024].

The Straits Times (2020, 13 March) 'Indonesia President Joko stokes speculation herbs can fight coronavirus', *The Straits Times*, Available from: https://www.straitstimes.com/asia/se-asia/indonesia-president-joko-stokes-speculation-herbs-can-fight-coronavirus [Accessed 8 July 2024].

Thelwall, M. (2008) 'Bibliometrics to webometrics', *Journal of Information Science*, 34(4): 605–21.

Thompson, C.M. (2015) *Vietnamese Traditional Medicine: A Social History (Vol 2)*, Singapore: NUS Press.

Thompson, C.M. (2017a) 'Selections from Miraculous Drugs of the South, by the Vietnamese Buddhist Monk-Physician Tuệ Tĩnh', in *Buddhism and Medicine: An Anthology of Premodern Sources*, New York: Columbia University Press, pp 561–8.

Thompson, C.M. (2017b) 'The implications of gia truyền: family transmission texts, medical authors, and social class within the healing community in Vietnam', *South East Asia Research*, 25(1): 34–46.

Thompson, L.C. (1988) *A Vietnamese Reference Grammar*, Honolulu, HI: University of Hawaii Press.

Touraine, A. (1971) *The Post-Industrial Society*, New York: Random House.

Touraine, A. (1977) *The Self-Production of Society*, Chicago, IL: University of Chicago Press.

Tovey, P., Easthope, G., and Adams, J. (eds) (2017) *Mainstreaming Complementary and Alternative Medicine: Studies in Social Context*, London, New York: Routledge.

Unschuld, P.U. (1988) 'Culture and pharmaceutics: some epistemological observations on pharmacological systems in ancient Europe and Medieval China', in *The Context of Medicines in Developing Countries*, Dordrecht, Boston, London: Springer, pp 179–97.

Uzzi, B. and Spiro, J. (2005) 'Collaboration and creativity: the small world problem', *American Journal of Sociology*, 111(2): 447–504.

Uzzi, B., Amaral, L.A., and Reed-Tsochas, F. (2007) 'Small-world networks and management science research: a review', *European Management Review*, 4(2): 77–91.

Van Dijk, J. (2020) *The Network Society*, London: SAGE Publications.

Van Dijck, J. and Poell, T. (2013) 'Understanding social media logic', *Media & Communication*, 1(1): 2–14.

van Eck, N.J. and Waltman, L. (2009a) 'Software survey: VOSviewer, a computer program for bibliometric mapping', *Scientometrics*, 84(2): 523–38.

van Eck, N.J. and Waltman, L. (2009b) 'How to normalize cooccurrence data? An analysis of some well-known similarity measures', *Journal of the American Society for Information Science & Technology*, 60(8): 1635–51.

van Eck, N.J. and Waltman, L. (2017) 'Citation-based clustering of publications using CitNetExplorer and VOSviewer', *Scientometrics*, 111(2): 1053–70.

van Eck, N.J., Waltman, L., Dekker, R., and van den Berg, J. (2010) 'A comparison of two techniques for bibliometric mapping: multidimensional scaling and VOS', *Journal of the American Society for Information Science & Technology*, 61(12): 2405–16.

van Es, K. (2017) *The Future of Live*, Cambridge, MA: Polity Press.

Vianello, R. (1985) 'The power politics of "live" television', *Journal of Film & Video*, 37(3): 26–40.

Vietnam National Archive (2020) 'Archive of Sai Gon Giai Phong Newspaper', Volume 4151 dated 17 November 1988, National Library of Vietnam, Available from: shorturl.at/hrwB7 [Accessed 8 July 2024].

VNExpress Online (2003) 'The dien chan method lacks scientific foundations', reprint from Lao Dong newspaper, Available from: https://vnexpress.net/phep-chua-benh-bang-dien-chan-chua-du-co-so-khoa-hoc-2255609.html [Accessed 8 July 2024].

Vraga, E.K. and Bode, L. (2017) 'Using expert sources to correct health misinformation in social media', *Science Communication*, 39(5): 621–45.

Vu, T., Nguyen, D.Q., Nguyen, D.Q., Dras, M., and Johnson, M. (2018) 'VnCoreNLP: a Vietnamese natural language processing toolkit', *arXiv preprint* arXiv:1801.01331.

Vu, V.H. (2020) 'An invention by a world-renowned doctor', *Dien Chan Viet Online*, Available from: http://www.dienchanviet.com/dien-chan/vu-van-hoi/bui-quoc-chau-nha-phat-minh-dien-chan [Accessed 8 July 2024].

Wade, G. (2000) 'The Southern Chinese borders in history', in G. Evans, C. Hutton, and K.K. Eng (eds) *Where China Meets Southeast Asia: Social & Cultural Change in the Border Regions*, New York: Palgrave Macmillan, pp 28–50.

Wahlberg, A. (2006) 'Bio-politics and the promotion of traditional herbal medicine in Vietnam', *Health*, 10(2): 123–47.

Wahlberg, A. (2007) 'A quackery with a difference – new medical pluralism and the problem of "dangerous practitioners" in the United Kingdom', *Social Science & Medicine*, 65(11): 2307–16.

Wajcman, J. (2015) *Pressed for Time: The Acceleration of Life in Digital Capitalism*, Chicago, IL: University of Chicago Press.

Waldstein, A. (2010) 'Popular medicine and self-care in a Mexican migrant community: toward an explanation of an epidemiological paradox', *Medical Anthropology*, 29(1): 71–107.

Waltman, L., Van Eck, N.J., and Noyons, E.C. (2010) 'A unified approach to mapping and clustering of bibliometric networks', *Journal of Informetrics*, 4(4): 629–35.

Wang, W., Chen, R.R., Ou, C.X., and Ren, S.J. (2019a) 'Media or message, which is the king in social commerce?: An empirical study of participants' intention to repost marketing messages on social media', *Computers in Human Behavior*, 93: 176–91.

Wang, Y., McKee, M., Torbica, A., and Stuckler, D. (2019b) 'Systematic literature review on the spread of health-related misinformation on social media', *Social Science & Medicine*, 240: 112552.

Watts, D.J. (1999) 'Networks, dynamics, and the small-world phenomenon', *American Journal of Sociology*, 105(2): 493–527.

Watts, D.J. and Strogatz, S.H. (1998) 'Collective dynamics of "small world" networks', *Nature*, 393(6684): 440–2.

We Are Social (2023) 'Digital 2023: your ultimate guide to the evolving digital world', Available from: https://wearesocial.com/digital-2023 [Accessed 8 July 2024].

Weisz, G. (2006) *Divide and Conquer: A Comparative History of Medical Specialization*, Oxford: Oxford University Press.

Wellman, B. (2001) 'Physical place and cyberplace: the rise of personalized networking', *International Journal of Urban & Regional Research*, 25(2): 227–52.

Whyte, S.R., Van der Geest, S., and Hardon, A. (2002) *Social Lives of Medicines*, Cambridge: Cambridge University Press.

Wohlgemuth, J. and Matache, M.T. (2014) *Small World Properties of Facebook Group Networks, Complex Systems*, 23(3), Available from: https://www.complex-systems.com/abstracts/v23_i03_a01/ [Accessed 30 August 2024].

Wootton, J.C. (2005) 'Classifying and defining complementary and alternative medicine', *Journal of Alternative & Complementary Medicine*, 11(5): 777–8.

World Health Organization (2012) *The Regional Strategy for Traditional Medicine in the Western Pacific (2011–2020)*, Manila: WHO Regional Office for the Western Pacific, Available from: https://iris.who.int/handle/10665/137517/discover [Accessed 8 July 2024].

World Health Organization (2013) WHO Traditional Medicine Strategy: 2014–2023, Available from: https://www.who.int/publications/i/item/9789241506096 [Accessed 23 May 2023].

World Health Organization (2023) 'Where we work', Available from: https://www.who.int/westernpacific/about/where-we-work [Accessed 8 July 2024].

Wu, A.X. and Taneja, H. (2021) 'Platform enclosure of human behavior and its measurement: using behavioral trace data against platform episteme', *New Media & Society*, 23(9): 2650–67.

Yang, Y., Wu, M., and Cui, L. (2012) 'Integration of three visualization methods based on co-word analysis', *Scientometrics*, 90(2): 659–73.

Zhang, E.Y. (2007) 'Switching between traditional Chinese medicine and Viagra: cosmopolitanism and medical pluralism today', *Medical Anthropology*, 26(1): 53–96.

Zhao, Y. (2018) *An Investigation of Autism Support Groups on Facebook*, doctoral dissertation, The University of Wisconsin-Milwaukee, Available from: https://dc.uwm.edu/cgi/viewcontent.cgi?article=2968&context= etd [Accessed 8 July 2024].

Zuckerberg, M. [Mark] (2016, 6 April) 'Today we're launching Facebook Live for everyone – to make it easier to create, share and discover live videos' [Facebook status update], Available from: https://www.facebook. com/zuck/posts/10102764095821611 [Accessed 8 July 2024].

Index

References to figures appear in *italic* type; those in **bold** type refer to tables.